NEURON STRUCTURE OF THE BRAIN

NEURON STRUCTURE
OF THE BRAIN

G. I. Poliakov

HARVARD UNIVERSITY PRESS
Cambridge, Massachusetts
1972

TT 70—50127

Prepared under the Special Foreign Currency Program of
The National Library of Medicine,
National Institutes of Health, Public Health Service,
U.S. Department of Health, Education, and Welfare,
and published for
THE NATIONAL LIBRARY OF MEDICINE
Pursuant to an Agreement with
THE NATIONAL SCIENCE FOUNDATION, WASHINGTON, D.C.
by
THE ISRAEL PROGRAM FOR SCIENTIFIC TRANSLATIONS,
JERUSALEM, ISRAEL

Copyright © 1972
By the President and Fellows of Harvard College
All Rights Reserved

Translated from Russian by P. Robinson, M.D.
Edited by T. Pridan, M.D.
ISRAEL PROGRAM FOR SCIENTIFIC TRANSLATIONS

Library of Congress Catalog Card Number 76-170287
SBN 674 60815 1

Printed in Jerusalem by Keter Press
Binding: Wiener Bindery

Table of Contents

	Page
INTRODUCTION	1

CHAPTER I. Reflex Mechanisms of the Brain
1. Organs of signalling activity 4
2. Fundamental subdivision of the nervous system 7
3. The coordinating mechanism 17
4. The analyzing-coordinating mechanism 29
5. Systems of analyzers 35

CHAPTER II. Regulation, Control and Direction in Animal Organisms
1. Presentation of the problem 40
2. Functional significance and interactions of various reflex mechanisms differing in their degree of development 41
3. Autoregulation and regulation 48
4. Autocontrol and control 49
5. General characteristics of autodirection and direction 52
6. Autodirection ("restricted," or automatic direction) 54
7. Direction proper ("free," or voluntary, and automatized (automatic)) . . 55
8. Psychophysiological aspects of the mechanism of direction 64
9. Interrelations of the functions of autoregulation, autocontrol and autodirection from the evolutionary point of view 68

CHAPTER III. The Neuron Network
1. Origin and differentiation of the neuron network 71
2. Progressive differentiation of neurons 73
3. Special transmitting neurons and their significance in reflex activity . . . 76
4. Forms of contacts and functional interrelations of neurons 83

CHAPTER IV. The Basic Pattern of Transmissions in the Neuron Network
1. The central transmitting structure in analyzers 91
2. Central nervous apparatuses of perception and impression 97
3. The structural basis of localization of cerebral cortical function 102
4. General scheme of interconnections between various levels of transmissions in analyzers 109

CONCLUSION	118
LIST OF ABBREVIATIONS	122

INTRODUCTION

The purpose of this monograph is to present some aspects of the origin, development, differentiation and specialization of reflex mechanisms in animals.

The structure of the brain as an organ interpreting the environment and directing the organism's reaction and behavior accordingly has played an increasingly important role in research and has been the subject of detailed experimentation. Further enlightenment in this field undoubtedly depends on the accumulation of relevant experimental data and on new information on the ultrastructure of the brain obtained with the light or electron microscope to reveal the interrelation between each of its constituent elements.

As more and more data have come to light, the need to interpret them has become increasingly important. Here an attempt has been made to correlate available data on the anatomy, physiology and evolution of the nervous system with results of more recent experimental methods reproducing physiological systems in vitro. At present, discussion must naturally be limited to hypotheses which help to clarify the general pattern of brain structure. Comparisons made between living and technical systems have usually been limited to the simplest models of the reflex arc or a single neuronal unit. When more complex CNS mechanisms were studied (such as models of a conditioned reflex), the actual analysis of these mechanisms was, in most cases, replaced by general schematic procedures, which by no means reflected the full real complexities of CNS structure. In spite of the undoubted value of these experiments on a simple cybernetic plane, the neuromorphologist is forced to acknowledge that they represent more of the cybernetic aspect than an exact knowledge of the brain.

In the first chapter a range of problems is examined; the queries raised vary in complexity and are set out in a certain order related to animal evolution, with reference to a basic plan of activating reflex mechanisms. At this stage it should be stressed that we did not base our concept of brain structure on the accepted anatomical division, but rather applied a new principle of functional localization; this is examined in detail in Chapter II.

In correlating the various stages of differentiation of animal reaction during the processes of evolution with alterations in neuronal structure, we integrated the relation of the three main functions which determine all possible adaptation mechanisms of the organism: regulatory function, control and direction, the last including autoregulation, etc. [autonomous nervous system functions].*

---

* In our article "Problema regulyatsii, kontrolya i upravleniya v neirofiziologicheskom aspekte" (Problems of Regulation, Control and Direction in the Neurophysiological Aspect), published in the book "Problemy kibernetiki," No. 11, 1964, we used the terms self-regulation and regulation, self-control and control, self-direction and direction. In the present monograph we have substituted the prefix "auto" for "self" so that our definitions may be differentiated more precisely from the interpretations of these terms used mainly in the psychological literature. The meaning remains unchanged.

To confirm our theory as stated above, our aim is to demonstrate that the morphological structure together with the functional aspects studied provide a feasible neurophysiological mechanism responsible for active orientation of the organism in relation to the environment, both external and internal, including analysis of signalization systems and appropriate responses. These reactions will then explain the mechanism of reflex response at all stages of evolutionary development. Further on it will be explained how the individual (topographic) pattern of the accurately delineated reflex mechanism for each of the given functions is determined, and how it is related to the corresponding neuron complexes and their interrelationships.

To avoid misunderstandings, it seems necessary to make the following proviso.

We could not find exact definitions for the terms "regulation," "control" and "direction" in the relevant literature, but arrived at our understanding of these functions exclusively through logical analysis of the reflex mechanisms in the animal organism. We consider these to be neurophysiological functions, brought about by absolute rules of inherent self-organizing systems.

It must be stressed that in the interpretation which follows, we consider the function of direction, along with the most complicated forms of analytical-synthetic processing of all information received by the organism, to be the highest expression of reflex activity (higher nervous activity, according to Pavlov's definition). We relate this function to the most highly organized parts of the central nervous system and ascribe the functions of regulation and control (according to our understanding of these definitions) to the lower levels of analyzers, considering them as being auxiliary to the main functional control which is recognized as the true organizer of all planning and direction of behavior. Our definitions of regulation and control thus differ from those generally accepted. We consider the manifestations of higher nervous activity in man, which on the psychological plane are often designated as regulation and control, as different forms of expression of the function of direction. In this respect we are more in agreement with those representatives of the cybernetic trend, who in determining the tasks of this trend, prefer to speak expressly of control function.

Chapters III and IV deal with the development of the system of neurons and the general pattern of neuronal structure and transmission in the CNS. We claim that a single common principle of general significance is responsible for the structure of all animal nervous systems from the simplest to the most complicated. According to this principle, any neuron, acting as the basic unit of the transmission process, is responsible for the collection and distribution of impulses passing through it, i.e., it fuctions as a physiological unit which fulfills the tasks of certain forms of analysis, synthesis and selection (filtration) of crossing impulses on the nerve cell level. This rule, which applies to all stages of evolution, at all levels of the nervous system, has enabled us to project a general pattern of successive differentiation of organization of neuronal transmissions, from the primitive neurons of the lower multicellular organisms to the most highly differentiated brain of the higher vertebrates and man.

With reference to the general nature of CNS structure, we will discuss here in greater detail the problem of rational classification of the cerebral cortex into different zones (anatomical areas and zones), depending on their function. The classification of cortical areas as delineated in this work has been confirmed by extensive long-term experience of clinical observations of cortical injuries.

The theories set out in this book are actually only working hypotheses, and are naturally subject to discussion. A thorough acquaintance with these theories may be of interest to a variety of specialists — not only neurologists, neuroanatomists, neurophysiologists and clinicians but also psychologists, pedagogues, biologists, physicists, as well as all scientists studying experimental models of biological systems.

It is our belief that the material presented may also assist in clarifying the philosophical concepts of the structure of the brain as an organ registering all aspects of environmental stimuli and processing them in the human and animal consciousness.

In Chapter IV we review more fully the mechanism's reflex activity in involving signalling systems, and the interstimulation of neurons, as an anatomical-physiological basis for registering and interpreting information in the cerebral cortex; in fact we stress that this is the underlying anatomical entity which functions as the interpreter of changes in the environment and regulates the organism's reaction to it. We also consider it of value to integrate into our concept of brain structure and function the known facts of evolutionary transitions in structure which have enabled the brain gradually to perceive and interpret not only usual sensory stimuli but also complex abstract ideas.

We regard the data presented in this work as a blueprint for a future concept of the neuronal construction of the brain.

Chapter I

REFLEX MECHANISMS OF THE BRAIN

1. ORGANS OF SIGNALLING ACTIVITY

In the evolution of the animal world the nervous system has developed as an interacting complex of organs which provide a highly effective structure for the adaptation of an animal to alterations in its environment, with the aid of the signalling system and its activity. Unlike plants, which react with changes in their activity only to direct external influences, animals are able to react to more highly complex signalling systems. The various stimuli are perceived by the animal not only as physical or chemical effects on the organism, but also as signals which are interpreted as indicators of certain vital changes. Animals thus differ from plants in their capacity to perceive and convert particular information received as impulses into certain relevant responses.

The following three basic elements, linked with each other in a definite order in the reflex arc pathway (Figure 1), are regarded as the physical basis of signalling (impulse) activity:

Receptor cells of the sensory organs, registering stimuli and transforming them into nervous impulses;

nerve cells with their dendrites, participating in various transmissions of nervous impulses in the course of their transfer from the primary to the terminal link of the reflex arc;

effector cells, such as muscles or glands, i. e., elements which effect reflex responses of the organism to stimuli.

The basic elements of the nervous system — the neurons — emerge and develop in the evolution of the animal world as a special apparatus connecting receptors and effectors. These neurons are responsible

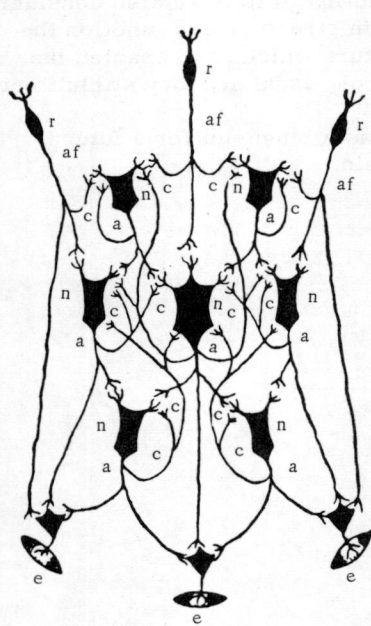

FIGURE 1. Diagram of the differentiated network of neurons:

r — receptors; af — peripheral sensory (afferent) fibers, carrying impulses from receptors to neurons; n — neurons; a — nervous fibers (axons) of nerve cells with dendrites (collateral branches — c), contracting with bodies of other nerve cells and their dendrites; e — effectors.

for determining the impulse significance of stimuli and for producing biologically expedient adaptive reactions.

The elements of the reflex arc are interconnected by special formations — the synapses. These structures will be described in greater detail in Chapter III. The subsequent transmission of impulses proceeds through the synapses, which receive and transmit from receptors to neurons, from one group of neurons to another, and finally from neurons to effectors.

In the course of development of the animal world, and in connection with the differentiation in interrelations with the external world, the mechanisms of the reflex impulse activity become very complicated. In their elementary form they are represented by a network of neurons (Figure 1), consisting of relatively simple combinations of receptors, neurons and effectors, which appear for the first time in lower multicellular organisms (Coelenterata).

This organization of the nervous system, on which its progressive differentiation is based, is already able to accomplish coordinated, i.e., regulated and biologically expedient, reflex responses to a stimulus.

Further differentiation of the system responsible for receiving impulses and activating effector reactions consists of the following elements.

The nervous mechanism of coordinated nervous activity, which emerges in the early stages of animal evolution, is capable of effecting regulated responses to a limited range of combinations of impulses with vital importance for the self-preservation and persistence of the species. However, this mechanism proves inadequate in cases where the organism is compelled to adjust to more complicated combinations of signalling systems. In themselves, these stimuli may not endanger the balance of the organism and may not originate directly from the sources of food; they simply inform the animal on the various changes in the environmental situation.

In subsequent stages of the evolutionary scale, the organism is able not only to carry out rapidly coordinated reflex responses to certain complex stimuli, but also to interpret in its more complicated reactions a space and time relationship between objects and events. This allows for a more differentiated orientation of external objects and their effect on the organism.

The development of more complicated mechanisms of perception and response have provided a means of constructing more complicated brain models for purposes of study. This evolutionary process has brought about a more highly developed signalling activity, or, according to another definition by Pavlov, to a higher stage of development of higher nervous activity.

Animals with a more primitively evolved signalling activity, capable of reacting in an orderly way only to a relatively narrow range of stimuli, may be compared in some way to living reflex self-adjusting "automatons." Organisms reacting to a wider range of stimuli, and presenting higher forms of reality perception, must interpret a considerably larger amount of incoming information from the environment. Compared with lower evolutionary orders, able to interpret a minimum of information, such organisms can be said to possess "surplus information" and are capable of "selecting" optimal solutions to various problems, including "deliberation" and "solution" of logical tasks. It is the evolvement of this quality that has led to the development of thinking beings.

With differentiations of receptions, the nature of responding actions has also become more differentiated. In the complicated fusion of conditioned and unconditioned reflexes which make up animal behavior, there is a continuing tendency to predominance of various forms of motivated co-ordinations perfected during life.

These changes in the manner of functional interrelations between the organism and the environment inevitably affect the structural organization of the sensory organs and nervous system and find their expression in the development of the analyzers.

Complicated neuronal linkages, of which the analyzers are composed, serve as the physical basis for a multitude of functional connections between separate signals and their combinations; in this manner the nature of relations between stimuli and the pattern of action response structured on this basis is determined.

In animal evolution the analyzers have developed as the most highly organized part of the neuronal structure of the brain, with the basic biological designation of fractional isolation of the separate signals, and the reaction to certain complexes of stimuli and their relations. As Pavlov pointed out, the analyzers are highly effective instruments for fine analysis and multifaceted synthesis of stimuli.

In the highest representatives of the vertebrates complicated networks of neuronal transmissions, of which the systems of analyzers are composed, are distributed in the various levels of the CNS (see Figure 7) and are adapted to the regulation of various components of reflex reactions, thus patterning the total behavior of the animal. The systems of analyzers which are distributed throughout the central nervous system are the most important part of brain structure; they play the role in the physiological unity of conditioned and unconditioned activity and thus ensure a balanced adaptation of the organism to the environment.

It should be pointed out that the differentiation in evolution of the physical components of the impulse activity mentioned above corresponds to some extent to the theories of McKey.* It is possible to find an analogy between the coordinating mechanism and the analyzers (see below) on the one hand and between the lowest and highest automatons on the other. The lower automatons (of the first order) work on an automaton-environment schedule. They are able to accomplish only the elementary function of direct "coding over" of external signals. The higher automatons (of the second order) possess an internal mechanism of confronting the external signalling system with their own programs of behavior; this mechanism is able to reproduce copies, models of certain features of objects and phenomena acting on the automaton, thus fulfilling the function of an analogue of the environment. As will be shown in the next section of this chapter, one of the significant differences between the analyzers and the coordinating mechanism is that the former provide the organism with a more complete and comprehensive orientation in the environment.

---

* See D.M. McKey. Development of the Concept of Action of Automatons. In "Automatons," edited by K.E. Shannon and J. McCarthy.

2. FUNDAMENTAL SUBDIVISION OF THE NERVOUS SYSTEM

Below is set out the general plan of the brain reflex mechanism in its different stages of differentiation, and the next chapter will deal with the relations of these mechanisms to the basic nervous functions of regulation, control and direction.

As already mentioned, in the evolution of the animal organisms possessing a nervous system there is an initial formation of a mechanism capable of carrying out coordinated reflex responses to stimuli. In other words, the elementary network of neurons (see Figure 1) has the basic function of a coordinating mechanism.

This organization is already clearly discernible in the earliest phases of animal evolution. Thus, the simplest unicellular organisms possessing only rudimentary sense organs and nervous system are in a position to accomplish well-regulated reactions, e.g., to use from their limited range certain definite, biologically expedient reflexes in a given situation, and inhibit reflexes hindering continuous activity.

In the course of progressive evolution the given mechanism of co-ordinated responses to stimuli becomes highly differentiated and specialized. Nevertheless, special groups of neurons responsible for this aspect of reflex activity can be formed in all representatives of invertebrates and vertebrates, both primitive and on a higher evolutionary scale.

In animals with bilaterally symmetrical bodies (including worms and higher animals), the coordinating mechanism forms a central axis of their central nervous system (Figure 2). In invertebrates it is connected with the thoracic ganglion (Figure 2A), by nerve cords in lower worms and by a chain of interconnected ganglia in annelids, crustaceans, arachnids and insects. It seems that at these stages of evolution the chain of ganglia distributed along the trunk carries out reflex functions that are analogous with the more complex coordinating activity mechanism in vertebrates.

In vertebrates this mechanism extends along the entire axial part of the central nervous system (the spinal cord and brainstem) (Figure 2B), occupying its central parts. Here it is important to mention the relatively direct character of interrelationships between receptors, neurons and effectors constituting the coordinating mechanism; one may assume that there are as many of these elements (but no more) as are essential for carrying out a particular coordinated reflext act.

The formation of analyzers is another development of this system which is of significance in the development of orientation of the organism in the environment and the far-reaching transformations of the entire sphere of its perception and relevant reaction. The physiological reason for the formation of these divisions of the entire reflex organization in the animal world is that the divisions enable the organism to perceive a multitude of "subsidiary" stimuli in a differentiated way, in addition to stimuli which are directly reprocessed by the coordinating mechanism, and ensure vitally important adaptations to environmental conditions. Thanks to the development of the analyzers, the organism receives a multitude of "inputs" and "outputs" to and from the periphery of the body in touch with the outside world. Thus, the organism is able to react in a selective way to the various signals, in a manner which functions beyond the scope of direct safety for the living system.

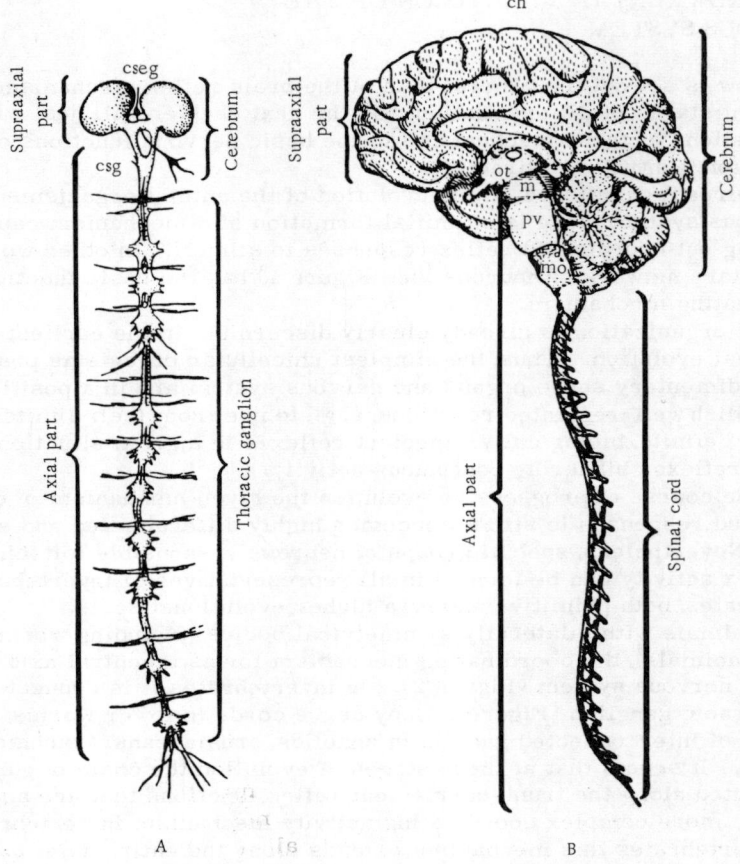

FIGURE 2. A — centralized ganglionic nervous system of a higher invertebrate (insect): cseg — cephalic supraesophageal ganglia; csg — cephalic subesophageal ganglia; B — central nervous system of the vertebrate (human brain): ch — cerebral hemispheres; ot — optic thalamus (diencephalon); m — mesencephalon (lamina quadrigemina and brainstem); pv — pons varolii; mo — medulla oblongata.

Pavlov defined analyzers as the complex links involved in transmission of nervous impulses, beginning with various sensory organs and ending with the brain. To clarify this function, he differentiated in each analyzer its peripheral and central (cerebral) end. In more highly organized representatives of the animal world the highest cerebral terminus of the system of analyzers is coordinated with the corresponding area in the cerebral cortex (see Figure 7).

The significant differences of the cerebral parts of the analyzer from the peripheral are as follows. Receptor elements of the sensory organs, and the peripheral sensory neurons directly connected with them (Figure 3, spn), are adapted exclusively to the purely "mechanical" discrimination of stimuli in accordance with their physical qualities (frequency, intensity, duration, etc.). The cerebral parts of the analyzers are specialized in central processes of analysis and synthesis of stimuli, not simply according to their physical and chemical parameters, but mainly according to their signal function as part of the life of the organism. Only on the basis of such mediatory processing of nerve signals are programs or formulas of responding actions and reactions of the organism developed.

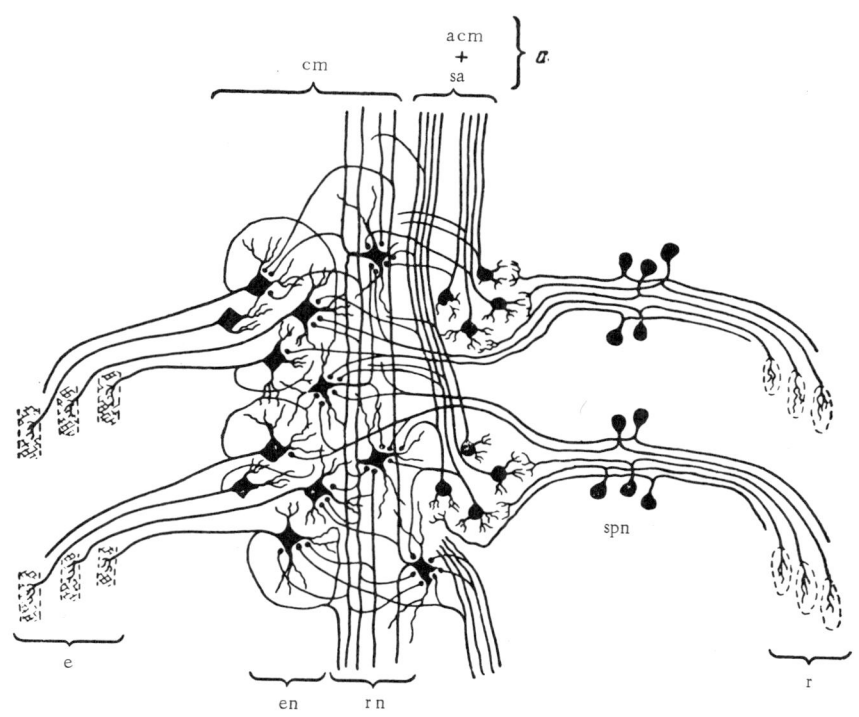

FIGURE 3. Diagram of transmitting arrangements of the CNS which form the coordinating mechanism (cm) and analyzers (a); the latter are composed of the analyzing-coordinating mechanism (acm) and systems of analyzers (sa); r — receptors; spn — sensory peripheral neurons present in ganglia of the cerebrospinal and cerebral nerves; rn — special transmitting neurons of the coordinating mechanism (reticular formation); en — effective (motor) neurons which innervate the effectors; e — effectors (skeletal muscles).

We include in the cerebral part of the analyzers only those groups of centrally transmitting neurons, with their interrelations, which could be considered as complementary superstructures to the transmitting neurons of the coordinating mechanism itself (Figure 3, see also Figure 18). In the centralized nervous system analyzers are represented as collections of neurons which are formed primarily in the "input" system of neuron networks, i.e., at points of transfer of impulses from peripheral sensory neurons into the coordinating mechanism. Analyzers represent an additional transmitting device, which is wedged in between the receptor sphere of the organism, and devices which directly organize its coordinated responses to stimuli.

From this topographic-anatomic correlation it follows that the basic physiological and biological designation of the analyzers is the organization of the sphere of reception of the organism itself. The cerebral parts of the analyzers participate in carrying out the interaction of various centripetal impulses incoming from the sensory organs. This type of interaction takes place even before the signalling impulses, transformed in a certain manner, are transmitted to the coordinated mechanism and are converted there into a specific corresponding effector activity.

The coordinating mechanism is concerned mainly with the reprocessing of relatively simple combinations of biologically adequate stimuli, which have not yet converged into more complicated physiological syntheses. The activity of the cerebral parts of the analyzers ensures the most highly organized central coordinations inside the receptor sphere itself, i.e., an analysis and synthesis of complexes of stimuli regulated in space and time and united in definite interrelated systems. Thanks to this complex mechanism the organism is able to orient and function as a complex differentiated entity in the external environment.

A useful illustration of this type of coordination, formed in the sphere of receptions of the organism, may be given by the results of the well-known experiments of Stratton,* using eyeglasses provided with lenses that give an inverted picture. After only a few days, complete reorientation in the environment is accomplished in the subject tested, and a normal perception of objects is established.

In organisms possessing developed analyzers, all reflex responses appear to undergo a special adaptation process through the prism of all processes of analysis and synthesis occurring in each case.

In the sphere of interrelations between the organism and the environment, the functional possibilities inherent in the coordinating mechanism itself are extremely limited. This reflex device is only suitable for the realization of separate, more or less elementary adaptations to relatively narrow distribution areas of life. The analyzers considerably extend the limits of adaptative possibilities of the organism.

Reactions achieved with the help of the coordinating mechanism are to a certain degree of a "transient" nature, each moment correlating the physical parameters of stimuli (their intensity, duration, frequency, etc.) with the physiological parameters of relatively simple reflex arcs.

The functional potentialities of the cerebral parts of the analyzers are much greater than those of the coordinating mechanism; thanks to their more complicated neuronal organization, they develop indispensable conditions not only for the synthesis of various reactions occurring at a given moment, but also for the functional connections of reactions in time. In other words, in the cerebral parts of the analyzers there is not only a direct correlation of the type of action of stimulus, and the nature of corresponding effector response at any moment, but there is also a complicated mediation of activity which occurs at a given moment, correlating with results of reflex actions performed earlier.

Analyzers apparently represent a more highly specialized instrument of reflex image of the environment as a complex and interrelated entity. Because of these analyzers, the organism is in a position to adapt itself to an increasingly greater number of variable combinations of stimuli.

---

* G. M. Stratton. Vision without Inversion of Retinal Image. — Psychol. Rev. No. 4. 1897.

The development of analyzers in the animal world has thus brought about a differentiated physical basis on which the continuity of individual experience is patterned. The potential of the organism to "foresee" probable consequences of its actions is increased accordingly. As will be shown below, particular formations of the cortical type especially adapted to performing the most complicated reflex functions have developed in the cerebral parts of the analyzers.

The formation of analyzers is conditioned by a qualitative differentiation of reactions coordinating the organism with the outside world. The effect of the outer, as contrasted with the inner, environment of particular importance in the progressive development of the analyzers.

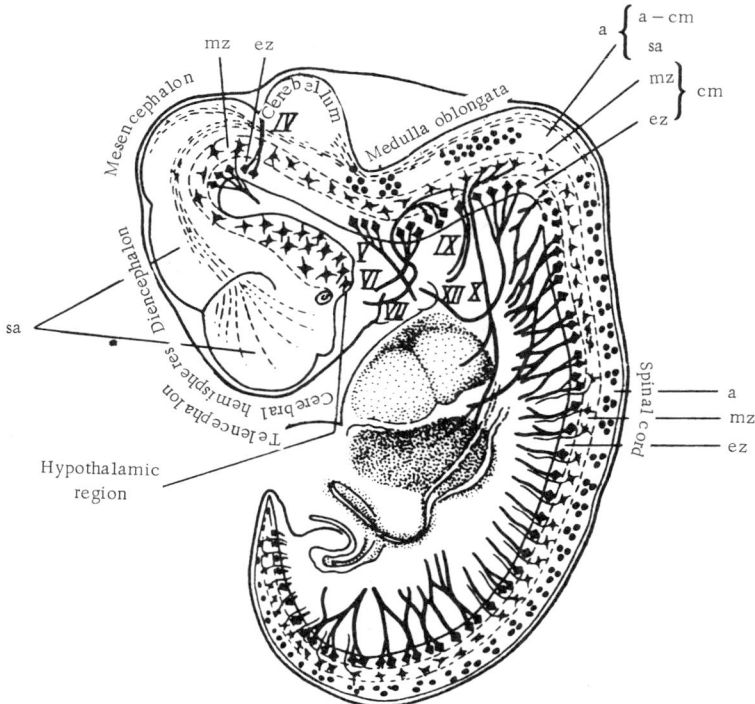

FIGURE 4. Diagram of the division of the CNS in a vertebrate. A human embryo at an early stage of development. Roman numerals denote the motor areas of the cerebral nerves; ez — zone of effector (motor) neurons with their exit points to the periphery; mz — zone of special transmitting neurons of the axial part of the CNS (reticular formation); mz + ez are included in the coordinating mechanism (cm); a — zone of analyzers, which later differentiate into the analyzer-coordinating mechanism (a–cm) and system of analyzers (sa); it may be seen that the reticular formation also extends into the supraaxial part of the CNS (see hypothalamic region of the diencephalon). The higher parts of the CNS — the cerebral hemispheres of the telencephalon — developed in their entirety from the zone of analyzers. (With partial use of the scheme of V. Gis and with reference to the latest research by G.P. Zhukova and T.A. Leontovich.)

The analyzers have appeared in the more highly developed invertebrates in a more rudimentary form; their central nervous representation here is in the more primitive brain (supraesophageal nerve ganglia in worms, insects, and crustaceans — see Figure 2A). However, only in vertebrates do the analyzers enter the decisive phase of their development, occupying more and more sections of the central and peripheral nervous system (Figure 4).

The chains of neuronal transmissions that constitute the analyzers are built on collections of neurons which make up a coordinating mechanism (see Figure 7). Guided more and more by the coordinating mechanism, the analyzers make use of its possibilities for more effective and adjustable adaptation of the organism to the variety of changing situations. With progressive development of the analyzers, the coordinating mechanism becomes more and more dependent on them, being transformed into a pliant instrument which carries out orders issued by the analyzers. In the course of evolution the coordinating mechanism, occupying a control position, becomes more and more superseded ("overgrown") by analyzer formations (Figure 5). At the same time, the analyzers become gradually independent from the coordinating mechanism from which they originally emerged.

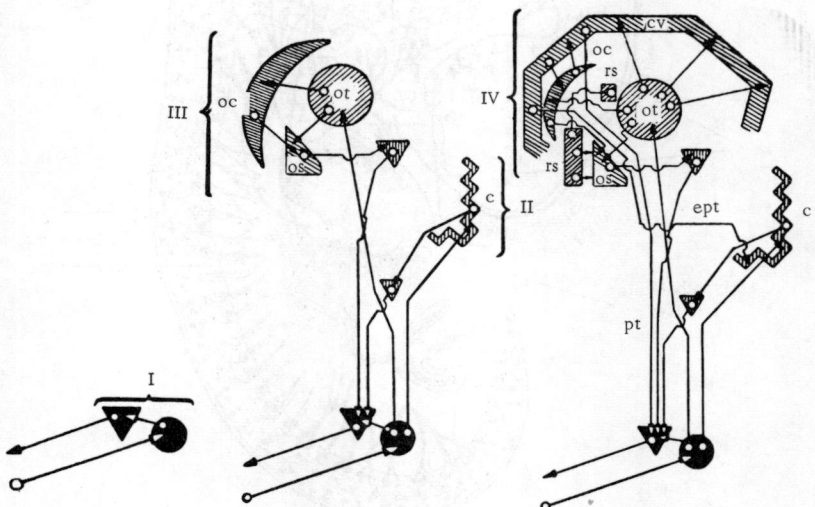

FIGURE 5. Diagram of "overgrowing" in the evolution of the coordinating mechanism of development of analyzers:

c — cortex of the cerebellum; ot — optic thalamus; oc — complex of phylogenetically older formations of the cortex; os — phylogenetically older part of the subcortical nodes of the cerebral hemispheres; rs — recent part; cv — the latest to appear in the evolution of vertebral formations of fully developed new cortex of the cerebral hemispheres; pt — pyramidal tract for the transmission of impulses of voluntary movements formed in the cortex to the reflex centers of the coordinating mechanism; ept — extrapyramidal path for the transmission of effect of the cerebral cortex on the cerebellar cortex. The lower reflex centers of the spinal cord and brainstem are represented by black circles and triangles. I corresponds to the coordinating mechanism, II to the analyzing-coordinating mechanism, III and IV to the two subsequent stages of progressive differentiation of higher (supraaxial) brain ends of the analyzer systems. (Somewhat modified sketch of N. A. Bernshtein.)

Thus, beginning with certain stages of evolution of animal organisms, the centralized nervous system* may be defined as the coordinating mechanism plus the aggregation of cerebral parts of the analyzers, closely interlinked. In this, the progressive increase in absolute and relative numbers of centrally transmitting neurons in the analyzers, relative to the neurons of the coordinating mechanism, can be used as a standard for measuring the level of neuron organization. On the relative-evolutionary plane two main divergent directions in the differentiation of the analyzer structure can be distinguished — representing two consecutive stages of their development — which complement each other and are included in a uniform functional architecture.

At the lowest stage of development, formed relatively early during phylogenesis, one can detect those formations of analyzers which are arranged at different levels of the axial part of the CNS and which are closely interconnected with elements of the coordinating mechanism. Those collections or groups that ensure further differentiation and expansion of the coordinating resources of the organism are designated here the analyzer-coordinating mechanism (see Figure 5 II). The latter is thus formed as a result of superimposition of the coordinating mechanism by elements of the analyzers.

The cephalic subesophageal nodes (see Figure 2A) are considered as an embryonic homologue of the analyzing-coordinating mechanism of the vertebrates, in which this mechanism is already distinctly formed. However, in the lower vertebrates (Cyclostomata) the basic mass of the central transmitting neurons can still be attached to the coordinating mechanism, whereas in fishes there is a rudimentary development of an analyzing-coordinating mechanism in the zones of all analyzers (Figure 6).

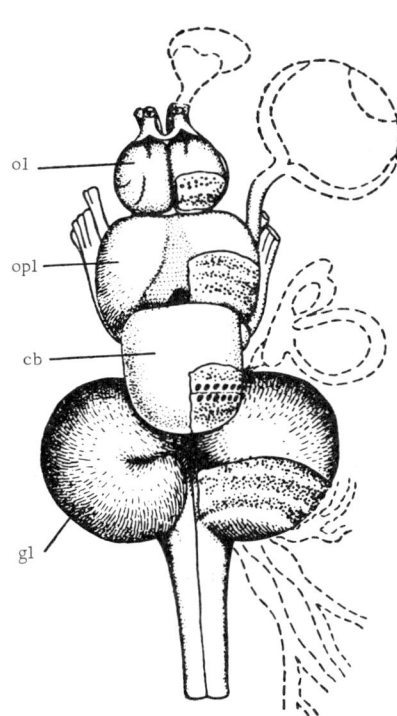

FIGURE 6. Diagram of the brain of a fish (carp) showing the relationships in the development of the cerebral parts of the various analyzers:

ol — olfactory lobe (prosencephalon); opl — optic lobe (mesencephalon); cb — cerebellum; gl — gustatory lobe of the medulla oblongata. On the right are sketched the transverse sections through the various parts of the brain to illustrate their structure according to the cortical type. (With partial use of Gerrik's figure.)

The highest degree of development of analyzers, which can be described as the greatest constructive achievement of living nature, is represented by systems of analyzers in the strict sense. The latter, as already mentioned,

---

* By centralized nervous system we understand the nerve ganglia in invertebrates and the central nervous system in vertebrates.

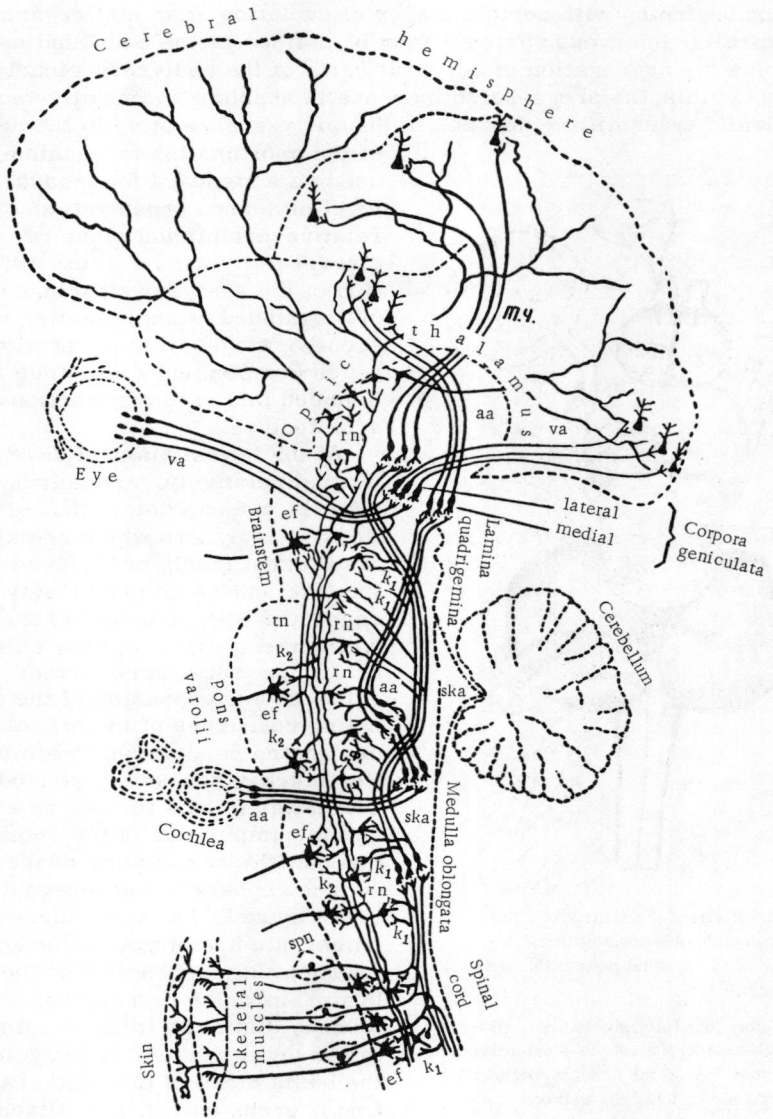

FIGURE 7. Diagram (of the contours of a human brain) of the main systems of analyzers and their connections with the coordinating mechanism. Depicted are the sensory organs, neuronal transmissions in the proximate and distal subcortex, and the cortical zones of analyzer systems:

va — system of visual analyzer; aa — system of auditory analyzer; ska — systems of skin and kinesthetic analyzers; spn — sensory peripheral neurons of ganglia of the cerebrospinal and craniocerebral nerves; ef — motor (effector) neurons of the spinal cord and brainstem; rn — transmitting neurons of the reticular formation (ef + rn — coordinating mechanism); K_1 — ramifications along the analyzer system to reticular and effector neurons; K_2 — terminal ramifications of reticular neuron axons connected with effector neurons. (With partial utilization of our 1959 scheme.)

are formed by complicated chains of transmissions (Figure 7) which extend throughout the CNS and connect the receiving surfaces of the sensory organs with the higher cerebral ends of the analyzers, representing the phylogenetically most recent supraaxial parts of the cerebrum (see below). The systems of analyzers are separated spatially from the analyzing-coordinating mechanism.

Manifestations of reflex activity, in the realization of which both coordinating and analyzing-coordinating mechanisms participate, are included here in a single common group of reflex coordinations. Both those mechanisms contained in the axial part of the CNS are jointly responsible for the physiologically regulated responses to stimuli; however, they are not yet sufficient for realizing all aspects of animal behavior.

Reflex coordinations which are carried out along the axial part of the CNS include the sum total of the particular reflex adaptations of the given organism to the conditions of its existence. They are separate "blocks" which are composed of important (vital) reactions inherited from ancestors, as well as those acquired in the course of individual life and connected with general orientation in the environment, provision of food, self-defense, continuation of the species, etc. Combinations of interconnected reactions programmed in the supraaxial part of the CNS constitute the total behavior of the organism.

In the evolution of vertebrates it is possible to follow in great detail the differentiation of reflex coordinations in accordance with their ascendence along the axis of the CNS, in connection with the differentiation of functional interrelations between the cerebral parts of the various analyzers. The "inventory" of the effector activities of the organism (according to N.A. Bernshtein's definition) becomes more enriched in phylogenesis as well as in ontogenesis.

The systems of analyzers interact with those parts of the neuron structure which have been differentiated most recently in the course of progressive evolution, reaching the highest structural and functional perfection and possessing the most highly developed adjustment mechanisms.

The systems of analyzers begin to be formed clearly in those vertebrates which have completed the transition from living in a more even aqueous environment to a more varied terrestial one (amphibians, reptiles). These formations reach peak development in structural and functional differentiation in higher mammals, particularly in man.

In contrast to the coordinating and analyzing-coordinating mechanisms, the highest cerebral ends of the analyzer systems exceed the limits of the axial parts of the centralized nervous system, forming its supraaxial part. The latter consists of a collection of "pure" neuron-analyzers with their interrelations, while in the axial part the analyzer-neurons closely adjoin the neurons of the coordinating mechanism (Figure 8).

In the higher invertebrates the supraaxial part represented by the cerebral supraesophageal nerve ganglia already mentioned (see Figure 2A) is relatively little developed. In vertebrates it is formed mainly in the telencephalon, which later develops into the cerebral hemispheres (see Figures 2B and 4), with their differentiation into cortical and subcortical formations (Figure 5) which arise during the phylogenesis of the higher vertebrates (mammals).

Reptiles, which are well adapted to terrestrial life, are capable of a more differentiated perception of external influences and of a more differentiated activity of parts of their body as compared with amphibians. For this reason they are the first among the vertebrates to display not only more finely processed axial mechanisms of reflex coordinations, but also a more precisely expressed differentiation of the supraaxial part of the CNS of the cortical and subcortical structure.

In the highly developed vertebrates (mammals) the highest cerebral ends of the system of analyzers are presented by formations of the fully developed cerebral cortex (see Figure 24) that are phylogenetically more recently separated and display the most elaborate differentiation into layers (see Figure 19D). These parts of the brain form a morphological groundwork on which a complicated mosaic pattern of stimulatory and inhibitory impulses is projected, originating from various complex and combined stimuli (objects) on the receptor surfaces of the sensory organs. The highest level of development and perfection in the organization of cortical formations in mammals is achieved in the primates, particularly in man.

It is precisely with these structures of the brain, the basic functional task of which is the identification of the signal significance of the multiform combinations of stimuli, rapidly changing in time and space, that the reproduction of brain models is connected, i.e., images of objects, phenomena, situations and their concepts; on the basis of such models one can program functions of various degrees of complexity in relation to the outside world. The highest brain ends of the systems of analyzers, which provide the organism with the fullest, most comprehensive and regulated information on the environment, represent the physical basis of reactions that coordinate the organism as a whole in the most delicately balanced and differentiated manner with the external world. They play a decisive role in the integration of various reflex adaptations — both those inherited by the organism and those developed in the course of individual life.

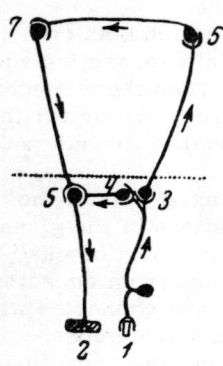

FIGURE 8. Diagram of transmissions in the axial and supraaxial parts of the CNS (compare with Figure 2B). The border between the two parts is marked by a dotted line:

1 — receptor; 2 — effector; 3 — neuron transmitting centripetal impulses to the supraaxial part of the CNS; 4 — neuron transmitting centripetal impulses to the level of the axial part; 5 — effector neuron; 6 — neuron transmitting centripetal impulses to the level of the supraaxial part; 7 — neuron of the supraaxial part carrying centrifugal impulses to the effector neuron of the axial part. It is seen that the supraaxial part contains only elements of analyzers, while in the axial part (3) these neurons are represented together with the neurons of the coordinating mechanism.

The following are the most important components that can be distinguished in the activity of the brain ends of the systems of analyzers:

a) determination of the signal significance of stimuli and systems of relations between impulses on the basis of analysis and synthesis;

b) programming of responding reactions to stimuli on the basis of integration of the total accumulation of signals with the biologically expedient use of the total available stock of reflex coordinations;

c) highest synthesis of the animal, exposed to the outer world, and vegetative factors, i. e., those connected with the internal environment, the activities of the organism in the process of its adaptation to the changing life conditions.

All those together make up behavior.

We shall now examine in greater detail some of the most important structural and functional features of the above-mentioned three basic parts of the nervous system and their interrelationships (see also scheme in Figure 21).

3. THE COORDINATING MECHANISM

The basic physiological task of the coordinating mechanism, as already mentioned, may be summarized as the process of producing formed responses to the direct action of certain combinations of vitally important stimuli.

The coordinating mechanism serves animal and plant reflexes of local significance, which can be said to be anatomically adapted to segmentary reflex arcs of the axial part of the central nervous system. These are: local defensive and adaptive reflexes, those connected with the intake and assimilation of food, simpler components of body balance in space and locomotion, in the form of cervical, vestibular and antigravitational reflexes (for instance, tendon reflexes), and also reflexes which aid in maintaining the tonus of skeletal muscles and reflexes of support and alternating movements of the extremities. The receptor fields of such reflexes are of relatively limited size and are localized mainly in those parts of the body and organs which participate directly in the realization of responses to stimuli (Figure 9).

The coordinating mechanism is seen to be adapted in the first place to coordinating groups of receptors and certain groups of effectors. With the evolutionary differentiation of the CNS, the activity of the coordinating mechanism is also further differentiated; as a result of a structural transformation taking place in this connection, the possibility is ensured of functional interrelations between the various reflex arcs along the total extent of the axial part of the CNS.

The first regulated reflex activity of any stage of differentiation — from the rhythmic beating of the umbrella of the jellyfish and crawling movement of the worm to the most refined movements of the human hand, eye and speech apparatus — is present in the form of an apparatus functioning on the "action-counteraction" principle, i. e., according to the type of linked functional agonist-antagonist pair. This principle was established by N. E. Vvedenskii and formulated by C. Sherrington as the rule of reciprocal innervation (Figure 10B). Such a physiological mechanism is most sensitive and able to accomplish coordinated movements, based on the simultaneous inclusion in the action of synergist effectors and the exclusion of counteracting effector antagonists, thanks to a strictly synchronized interaction of processes of stimulation and inhibition in both members of the linked pair. As a result of their fixed tension, the synergic muscles in this process act in a manner to curb any excess degree of freedom of mobility of the corresponding organ, thus permitting the latter to move in one specific direction.

There is reason to assume that the state of reflex activity is directly associated with the formation of the physiological mechanism of the linked function of a pair, both in the evolution of animal life, and in the course of individual development of the organism in intrauterine and extrauterine life.

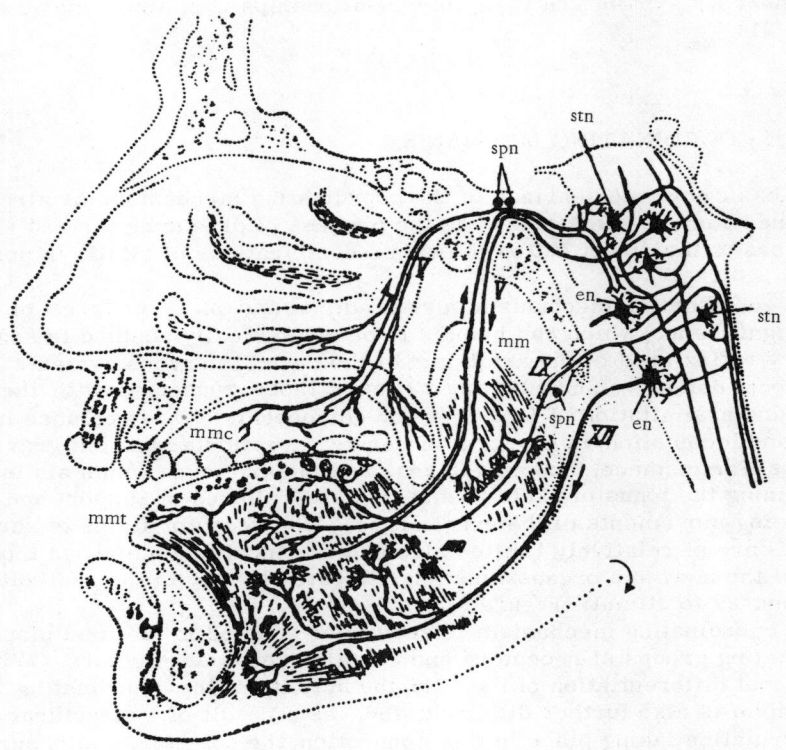

FIGURE 9. Diagram of the interrelations of elements concerned with reflex coordination of mastication, resulting from stimulation of the mucous membrane of the mouth and tongue by a certain food. The pertinent cerebrospinal nerves, transmitting the centripetal impulses, are marked with Roman numerals (see arrows):

mmt — mucous membrane of the tongue; mmc — mucous membrane of the oral cavity; mm — mastication muscles; spn — sensory peripheral neuron; stn — special transmitting (reticular) neuron; en — effector neuron. (With partial use of diagrams by various authors.)

At least two stages can be distinguished in the consecutive differentiation of interaction between receptors, neurons and effectors, leading to structural adjustment of the given mechanism.

In some more primitive multicellular animals there is apparently a simpler structure which still works on the principle of simple alternation of inclusion and exclusion of the same group of effectors (Figure 10A). It may be assumed that this activity also occurs during the rhythmic contractions and relaxations of the umbrella of the jellyfish, by means of which the animal moves. The umbrella contains a network of radial and circular cords of muscle fibers, contracting and relaxing synchronously as a result of the fact that the impulses of stimulation are transmitted throughout the nervous system of the jellyfish, registering and activating all effector elements of the body. Their exclusion follows the inclusion. Such a primitive structure still combines the physiological properties of a linked agonist-antagonist pair in the activity of one common group of effectors.

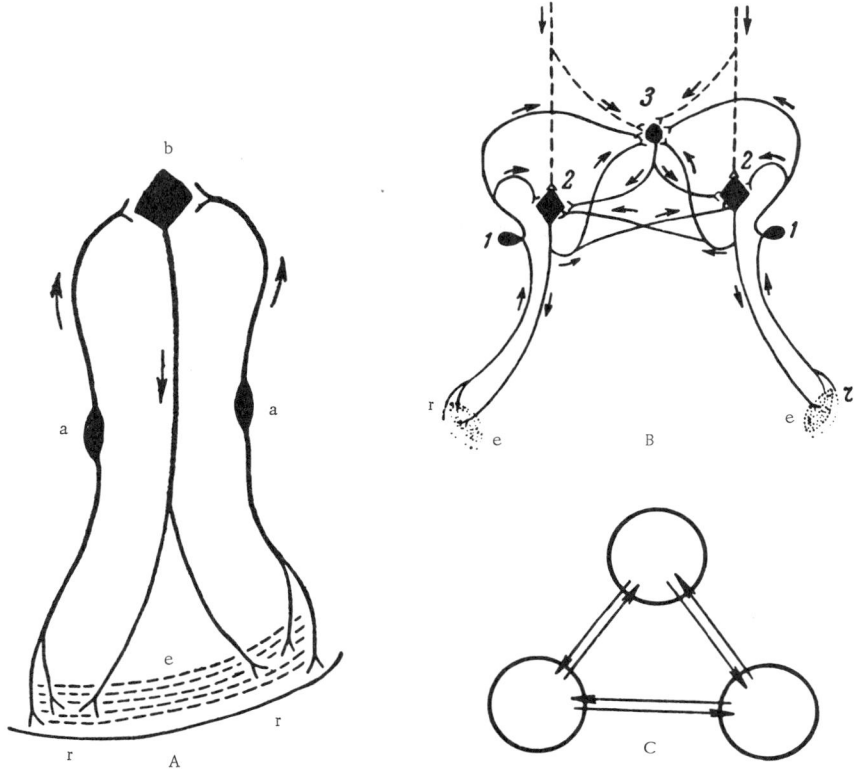

FIGURE 10. Three diagrams of coordinating apparatus:

A. Diagram of the simplest coordinating apparatus of a primitive multicellular organism: r — receptor; e — effector (muscular system); a — sensory neuron; b — neuron combining the functions of effector and transmitting elements.
B. Diagram of an elementary coordinating apparatus working on the principle of a linked functional agonist-antagonist pair: r — receptor; e — effector; 1 — peripheral sensory neuron transmitting centripetal (afferent) impulses from receptors to an effector (motor) neuron (2), as well as to a specially transmitting neuron with multiple dendrites (3); as presented in the diagram, the latter ends with ramifications of its nerve fiber (axon) on both effector neurons. Elements of the reverse connections are presented by lateral and reverse collaterals of the axons of effector neurons. Directions of movements of nerve impulses are shown by arrows. Descending (centrifugal) conductors, reaching with their end branches both the effector and the specially transmitting neurons, are indicated by dotted lines.
C. Geometrical diagram of bilateral functional interactions among the three central neurons of the elementary coordinating apparatus as an autoregulating system.

The structural separation of the two effector members of the pair, connected with corresponding transformations in the receptor as well as the neuron organization, is clearly represented in the lower worms (Figure 11). These animals, adjusted to the more complicated conditions of terrestrial life, are capable of carrying out more varied locomotor functions than the jellyfish. Two distinctly separate anatomical groups of muscle fibers, with different effects of function, are present in the muscular sac of these worms. One consists of circular muscle fibers, distributed parallel to the body axis, the other of longitudinal fibers. Contraction of the circular muscles results in elongation of the body, while contraction of the longitudinal muscles causes its shortening. Rhythmically coordinated movements of crawling are accomplished through the mechanism of alternating synchronization and activation of one group of muscles and inactivation of the other, i. e., according to the principle of reciprocally innervating relations between agonist and antagonist.

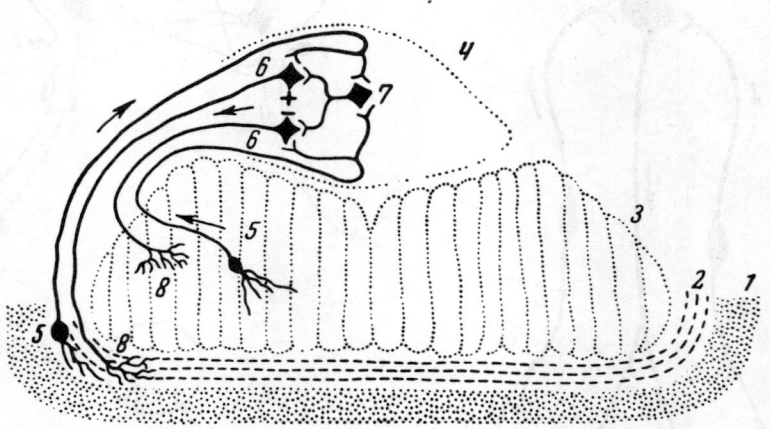

FIGURE 11. Diagram of the structure of a linked agonist-antagonist functional pair in a worm:

1 — dermal cover of the body; 2 — layer of circular muscles, elongating the body; 3 — layer of longitudinal muscles, shortening the body; 4 — nerve ganglion; 5 — peripheral sensory neuron; 6 — effector neuron; 7 — specially transmitting neuron; 8 — motor end in a muscle.

In animal organisms of complicated structure this principle is most distinct in a double (sympathetic and parasympathetic) innervation of all internal organs and systems (Figure 12). The functional relations between the two components of the autoregulating system have developed in these phylogenetically oldest physiological autoregulations, on which the biological activity of the body directly depends.

The synchronized interrelation between agonists and antagonists also serves as a basis for all coordinated motor activity whether voluntary or involuntary. In activities pertaining to interrelations of the organism with the environment, the mechanism of reciprocal innervation has become functionally more mobile than in activites concerned with internal autoregulations; the former involves a simultaneous and consecutively common activity of several different groups of skeletal muscles in various combinations.

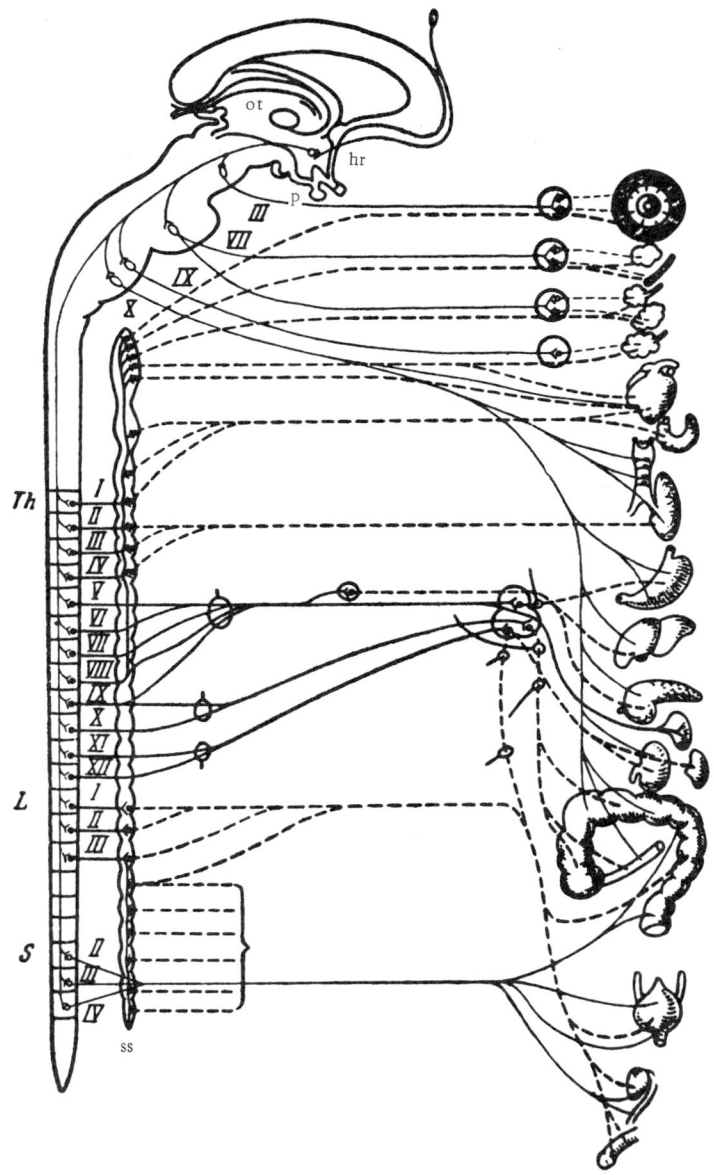

FIGURE 12. Bilateral autonomic innervation of internal organs. Fibers of the sympathetic nervous system reaching the organs are indicated by dotted lines; the parasympathetic nervous system is indicated by continuous lines. The diagram shows the lateral chain of sympathetic ganglia situated along the spinal column (ss) and the sympathetic ganglia and nerve plexuses in the area of the head and in the inner cavities of the body: ot — optic thalamus; hr — hypothalamic region; p — pituitary. The cranial nerves and roots of the corresponding segments of the spinal cord are marked by Roman numerals.

To understand the role of coordinating reflex action in the life of each organism, it is of interest to note the functional transformations observed in crossing sutures of tendons of agonist and antagonist muscles or of the nerves that innervate them (A. Bethe,[*] E. A. Asratyan[**] and others). It has been shown, for instance, that when flexor muscles of the extremities are connected with nerve centers of extensor muscles — and the extensor muscles themselves — to nerve centers of flexor muscles, both types of muscle at first function in an uncoordinated manner. In time, however, the physiological mechanism of synchronized activity of flexors and extensors on the agonist-antagonist pattern is resumed. It is especially interesting that in this case the biologically expedient use that the organism makes of its effector apparatuses in order to realize the various adjusting reactions is fully reestablished. Under particular conditions, such as before surgery, the organism responds with reactions adequate to the stimuli, regardless of the radical changes in relations between the nervous centers and the organs innervated by them. It is also interesting that the new coordinating relations have similarly proved to be effective in stimulations arising from higher parts of the CNS (upon stimulation of the cerebral cortex).

As to the special structural characteristics of the coordinating mechanism, we must comment as follows:

The linked agonist-antagonist pair could be regarded as the elementary coordinating mechanism, in some way as a physiological component of the entire coordinating mechanism. As seen in Figure 10B, the incoming part of the system described consists of a pair of receptor elements and the peripheral sensory neurons connected with them; these are strictly specialized for the function of carrying impulses from the receptor to the central neurons. The outgoing part is represented by a pair of corresponding effectors (striated skeletal muscles, smooth muscles of internal organs). The central part of the system thus presented, that which carries out the most responsible function, is formed by three elements — the central neurons. Together with both motor (effector) neurons which directly innervate the corresponding effectors it is essential for a third element, a particular neuron (intermediate, or inserted), to participate; this is regarded as a special transmitting neuron.

The three central neurons which participate in this combined mechanism form, as will be shown below (see Chapter II, Section 3), a central link in the autoregulating system, so interrelated that each can act on two other neurons and in turn is acted on by them (Figure 10B). The physiological mechanism of summation and interference of stimulations in nerve centers is conditioned by the interaction of impulses, circulating in a similar elementary section of the neuronal network. According to recent electrophysiological research (see Chapter III, Section 3), an active part in this process is ascribed to those neurons which we denoted as the "transmitting" ones. It has been shown, in particular, that these elements, as opposed to the effector (motor) neurons, are characterized by a very low excitability threshold and are capable of regenerating high-frequency rhythmic discharges of up to a thousand and more impulses per second in

---

[*] A. Bethe. Studien über Plastizität des Nervensystems. — Arch. ges. Physiol., p. 224. 1926.
[**] E. A. Asratyan. Fiziologiya tsentral'noi nervnoi sistemy (Physiology of the CNS). — Moskva, Izdatel'stvo Akademii Nauk SSSR. 1953.

response to a single afferent stimulus. Such a transformation of a single stimulus into high-frequency discharges is apparently of considerable significance in determining the functional state of effector neurons constituting a part of the central transmitting apparatus. The changes in excitability of effector neurons, determining critical points, or thresholds, and their transition from a state of excitation to a state of inhibition in a repeating cycle, depend directly on impulse transmission by special neurons.

There are grounds for assuming that no regulated reflex act could be realized by the action of effector neurons alone, i.e., without the cooperation of added special transmitting neurons. Elements of this kind, together with reverse collateral axons of effector neurons (Figure 10B), play a significant role in the distribution of afferent impulses among the corresponding groups of effector neurons, and also in the closure of links of cyclic circulations of impulses (see Chapter IV, Section 2) during the process of their progressive transmission of impulses from receptors to neurons.

Owing to a corresponding organization of interrelations among (a) peripheral neurons carrying impulses from receptors, (b) the effector neurons and (c) the special transmitting neuron, the last is able to participate in particular in the progressive and regressive connections of both reflex arcs, linked in a single paired functional system. In the presence of physiological parameters of all elements selected and coordinated among themselves, the special transmitting neuron appears as a fairly adaptable formation from the functional aspect, affecting the distribution of conditions of stimulation and inhibition in agonist-antagonist centers and regulating the reciprocal inclusion of some effectors and the exclusion of others.

In the activity of any coordinating apparatus the special transmitting neuron is an element responsible for the correlation, control and comparative evaluation of impulses acting simultaneously and consecutively and of the reactions caused by them in the effector ends of both reflex arcs.

Entering into the function of this element (as can be judged from the diagram in Figure 10B) is a correlation, according to the principle of reverse connection of signals, between an action and information on an action that is actually to be carried out.

Signals arising from the higher parts of the CNS, like the signals arising from the periphery, refer simultaneously to the executive elements of the reflex arc effector neurons, as well as to the special transmitting neuron (Figure 10B). This organization of interrelation between neurons allows for the autoregulating physiological system of the corresponding coordinating mechanism centers to become accessible to influences from the higher brain control centers.

There are several morphological proofs of this concept. Terminal ramification of fibers incoming from the periphery (centripetal), as well as fibers originating in the more highly located parts of the CNS (centrifugal), have been noted to reach not only the effector neurons but also the auxiliary transmitting neurons of the spinal cord and brainstem. This was shown to be the case in one of the main pathways of the CNS — the motor cortex (pyramidal tract), which is responsible for transmission of voluntary impulses and movements.

The combination of three central neurons (two effectors and one concerned particularly with transmission), constituting the basic unit of the coordinating mechanism, may be regarded as an apparatus which in view of its properties and effective possibilities seems to correspond to the principle of function of the most effective regulator. It may be assumed that like the latter, the system of bilateral interrelated neurons is capable of selecting and dealing with the optimal variants of functional conditions of the separate elements and their interrelations in a specific type of reaction.

The outline presented here may also be regarded as a basis for a general organization of all degrees of complexity of carrying out a temporary relation in which, with regard to both members of the linked functional pair, reflex arcs of conditioned and unconditioned stimuli are projected. Of principal interest is the fact that in outlines of experimental models of closure of a conditioned reflex, we find an analogue of a special transmitting neuron (Figure 13) together with elements of direct transmission of impulses, distributed along the pathway of both reflex arcs ("supported" and "supporting"). As was shown in a series of recently conducted electrophysiological investigations (G. Gasto,* A. Fessar** and others), the convergence of various afferent impulses onto the specially transmitting reticular neurons apparently plays a certain role in the realization of those components of the function of reflex arc closure which traverse the subcortical CNS levels. This outline could also be presented as the prototype of a "logical" mechanism, accomplishing a selection of a certain variant out of two or more possibilities.

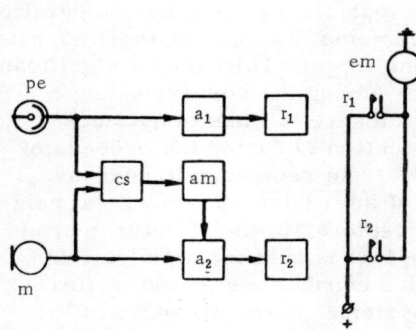

FIGURE 13. "Blueprint" diagram of a model of a conditioned reflex:

pe — photoelement; m — microphone; a — amplifier; r — relay; em — electric motor; cs — diagram of coordination system; am — accumulating mechanism. In this diagram the elements cs and am play the role of the special transmitting neuron, interposed between the two chains of direct transmission of impulses (pe — a_1 — r_1 and m — a_2 — r_2). (After L. P. Kraizmer, modified.)

In nervous systems in vivo a collection of special transmitting neurons forms a network (reticular formation) of the spinal cord and brainstem (Figures 3, 4 and 7). The collection of neurons of the reticular formation of the axial part of the CNS represents, at all stages of vertebrate evolution, a complex of intricately interrelated special transmitting neurons and is the most important integral part of local coordinating reflex apparatuses.

Neurons of reticular formations play the role of "selectors", distributing impulses coming from receptors, but also other parts of the CNS in various groups of effector neurons, placed on the same (or different) levels of the axial part of the CNS (Figure 14). It is to be noted that this very formation constitutes the original basis of the CNS to which, in the course of evolution, the complex system of analyzers is added.

---

[*] H. Gastaut. The Role of the Reticular Formation in the Production of Relative Reflex Reactions. In: "Reticular Formation of the Brain." [Russian translation. 1962.]

[**] A. Fessard. Analysis of Completion of Temporary Connections on the Level of Neurons. In: "Electroencephalographic Studies of Higher Nervous Activity." [Russian translation. 1962.]

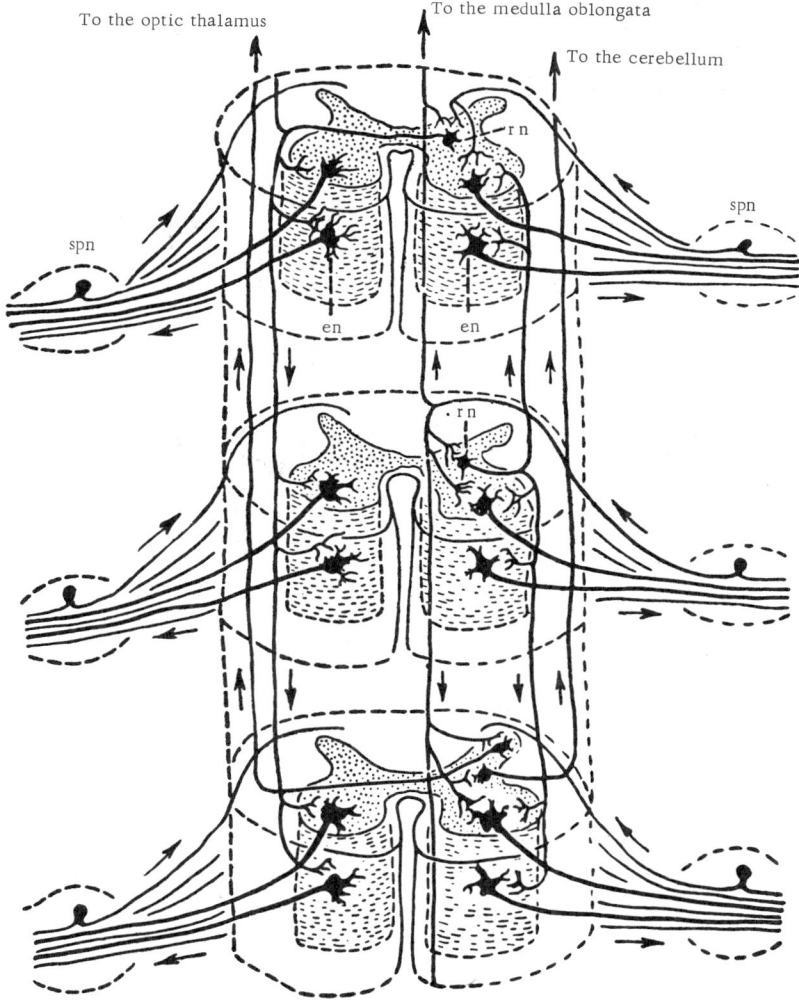

FIGURE 14. Diagram of intersegmentary connections of the coordinating mechanism. Depicted are three adjacent segments of the spinal cord:

spn — sensory peripheral neurons of intervertebral nodes; rn — neurons of the reticular formation distributing afferent impulses to different groups of effector (motor) neurons (en). The arrows show the direction of movement of the impulses. The elements of the coordinating mechanism are shown together with some conduction pathways, related to the analyzing-coordinating mechanism and to systems of analyzers (note arrows indicating cerebellum, medulla oblongata and optic thalamus).

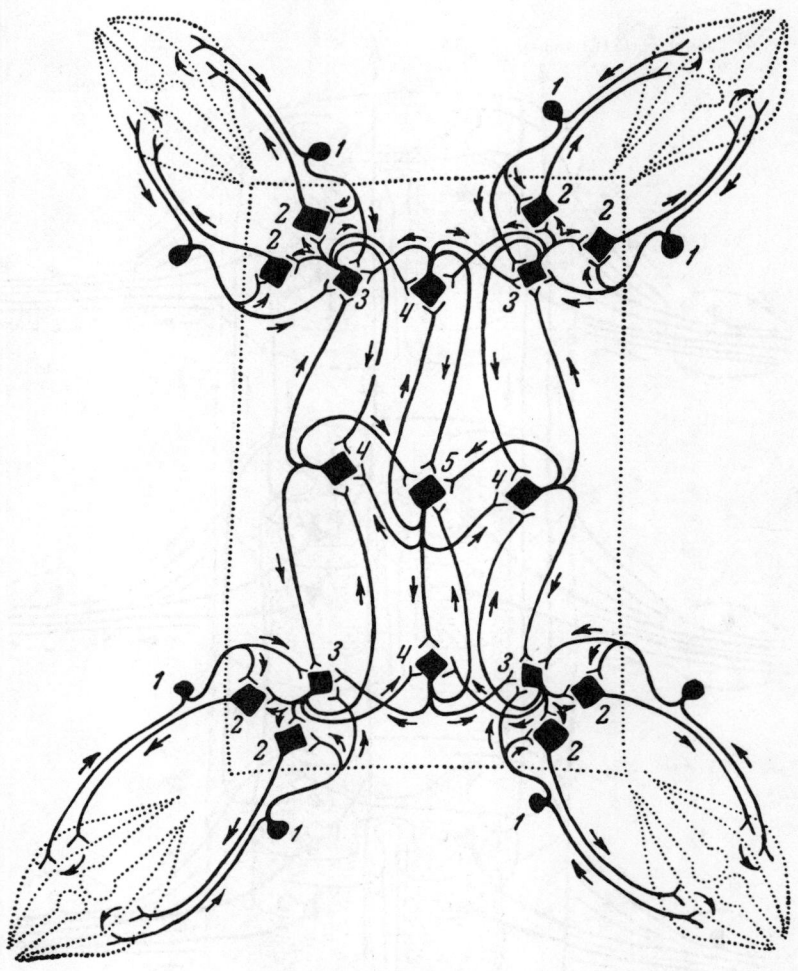

FIGURE 15. Diagram of the transmitting apparatus of a section of the coordinating mechanism serving coordinating movements of all four extremities:

1 — sensory peripheral neuron; 2 — effector neuron; 3, 4, 5 — special transmitting neurons. The central apparatus which innervates each "agonist-antagonist" pair belonging to one extremity includes a certain group of special transmitting neurons of the first order (3, compare with 3 in Figure 10B). Interaction of two "agonist-antagonist" pairs, related to the corresponding pair of extremities (both anterior and posterior limbs, right and left) is accomplished through the auxiliary group of transmitting neurons of the second order (4). Interaction of "agonist-antagonist" pairs related to all four extremities is accomplished by means of one additional group of special transmitting neurons of the third order, occupying a central position (5). All groups of special transmitting neurons indicated are functionally interrelated by closed circuits of circulation of impulses.

The following problem is of interest: how far can the differentiation of function of the coordinating mechanism proceed by means of its enrichment with networks of neurons and an increase in the interrelations of these neurons with effector neurons? In other words, to what degree can the "organized" possibilities included in the properties of the coordinating mechanism itself be realized without the additional participation of the analyzer and its reflex transmissions?

The diagram in Figure 15 depicts the differentiation in interrelations of the neuronal network in effecting locomotor activity of which a mammal is capable, in this case the drawing in of all four extremities for the coordinating and collaborating movements of walking, running, etc. To interpret this diagram, we may assume that the transmitting mechanism of the reticular formation is capable of encompassing and uniting, in a single reflex action, a larger or smaller number of separate "segment" reflexes along the CNS axis. The fact that a decapitated animal is still in a position to execute coordinated locomotor movements serves as physiological confirmation of such an assumption.

Groups of reticular neurons joined in a certain way along the total axial part of the CNS form a supersegmentary apparatus of the coordinating mechanism.

A study of the changes taking place in the CNS of vertebrates in the course of evolution leads one to conclude, at the same time, that the differentiation of neuronal networks has certain limitations. During further differentiation of reflex coordinations produced in connection with the development of analyzers, some supersegmentary parts of the coordinating mechanism, related to complex reflex acts, are gradually transformed into an integral part of the analyzing-coordinating mechanism.

The latest experimental-morphological studies of Zhukova and Leontovich* have shown that the reticular formation also exerts its affect on the phylogenetically oldest parts of the supraaxial zone of the CNS, located at the base of the brain. These zones, which are in fact direct extensions of the axial part of the CNS, include in particular the hypothalamic region of the mesencephalon (see Figure 4) and some of the oldest formations of the so-called semi-isolated cortex (according to the classification of I. N. Filimonov), together with the adjacent subcortical formations (see Figure 5, dsk). All structures indicated predominate in lower vertebrates in which the telencephalon is still not fully developed, and the cerebral hemispheres not yet present (Cyclostomata, fish).

In addition to the various segmental reflexes mentioned previously, the concept of "auxiliary control" of the coordinating mechanism includes autonomic nervous system activity. The reflex coordinations distributed along the axial part of the CNS, concerned with various vital functions and connected with pain responses to direct injury to body tissues, are concentrated in the coordinating mechanism itself (Figure 16). These reflex reactions are apparently represented only to a slight degree in the analyzing-coordinating mechanism. This may be deduced from the fact that local autonomic, as well as local defense, reflexes are maintained in the presence of intact segmental arcs and brainstem, and also in the central apparatus of transmissions and connections in the reticular formation itself.

---

* G. P. Zhukova and T. A. Leontovich. Osobennosti neironnoi struktury topografii retikulyarnoi formatsii u khishchnykh (Features of Neuron Structure and Topography of the Reticular Formation in Carnivores). — Zhurnal vysshei nervnoi deyatel'nosti, Vol. 14, No. 1. 1964.

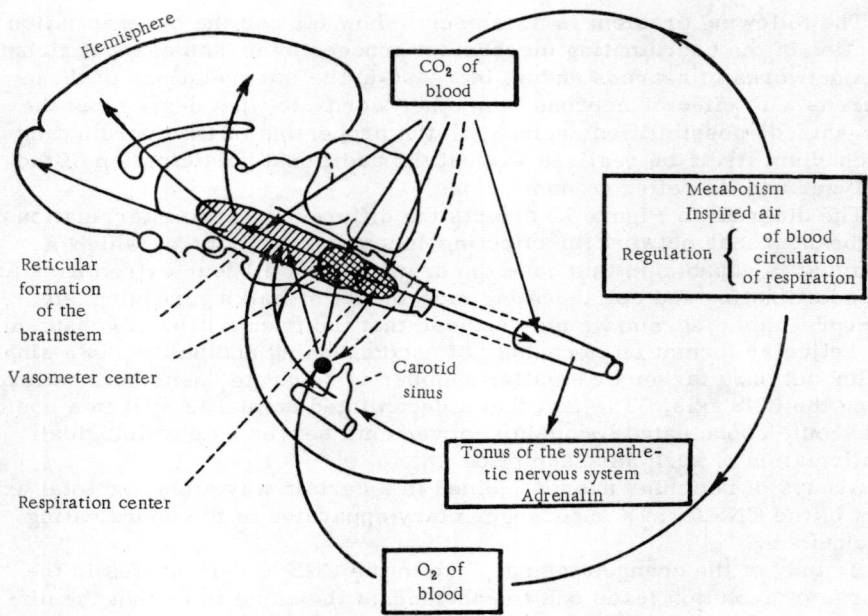

FIGURE 16. Diagram illustrating the localization of central representation of the autonomic functions of the organism (respiratory, cardiovascular) in the reticular formation of the brainstem. It depicts some autoregulatory physiological systems of the internal environment of the organism involved in the functional cycle under control of the reticular formation of the cerebrum and spinal cord. It also indicates the effects of the reticular formations of the brainstem on the proximal supraaxial brain (cerebral part), and the distal components of the CNS (spinal cord). Ascending effects of the reticular formations of the brainstem form one generalized, coordinated activated system. (After Dell and Bonvalle.)

    This type of reflex function in animals seems to include certain defense reflexes involving a change in the pigmentation of the skin related to alterations in coloration of the external background; the higher central representation of such reflex responses is apparently associated with hypothalamic function. The stages composing the reflex arc itself may be delineated as follows: the retina of the eye which receives the stimulus, the optic nerve, the hypothalamic nuclei; from there the impulses are transmitted in part to the autonomic centers of the brainstem, and in part through the pituitary to the endocrine glands which, together with the autonomic nervous system, control skin pigmentation. The particularly specialized functions of the coordinating mechanism must also include, for instance, in the frog, the retinomotor effects on the eye in response to exposure of the skin to light. Some investigators (D. A. Biryukov[*]) stress the significance of visual stimuli in the maintenance of the general skeletal muscle tone (phototonic function of the receptor section of the visual analyzer).

---

[*] D. A. Biryukov. Ekologicheskaya fiziologiya nervnoi deyatel'nosti (Ecological Physiology of Nervous Activity). — Leningrad, Medgiz. 1960.

Anatomically, the coordinating mechanism also includes the central gray matter lining the fourth ventricle of the brain and the Sylvian fissure, and extends into the hypothalamic nuclei of the mesencephalon (midbrain). This formation also consists of reticular-type neurons (G. P. Zhukova, 1964) and, from the physiological view may be considered mainly as the central representation of various autonomic autoregulating mechanisms of the organism. It must be assumed that the central gray matter of the brain, represented to a particularly marked degree in amphibians, is of great importance for the individual adaptations of organs and parts of the body to conditions governing their activity. The hypothalamic nuclei (see Figures 4 and 12) affect various aspects of the vital activity of the organism as a whole, including trophic, metabolic and various continuous processes of adjustment of living matter in cells and tissues.

Recently, morphological investigations have confirmed the theory that quite a significant part of the autonomic activity of the organism, in terms of a complex system of reflexes functioning to adjust to needs of the inner environment, is governed by the coordinating mechanism. It was proved that autonomic (sympathetic and parasympathetic) centers of the spinal cord and brainstem (Figure 16) as well as the central gray matter of the brain and the hypothalamic region, are formed from typical reticular neurons (Zhukova and Leontovich — see above), differing in their structural features from motor neurons, and neurons of which analyzers are composed (Figures 17 and 30).

Thus, it may be assumed that in the evolution of vertebrates the central nervous mechanisms transmitting signals arising from the internal environment of the organisms are not yet isolated to a major degree from the midst of the coordinating mechanism. This category of reflex processes occurring in the body itself could be connected only indirectly with the activity of the analyzers. Such a conclusion is consistent with the view shared by many physiologists, namely that interreceptions are represented to a much less pronounced degree in the cerebral cortex than incoming stimuli that are directly related to the analyzer systems.

4. THE ANALYZING-COORDINATING MECHANISM

As the heading indicates, this is a composite formation consisting of an evolutionally old part (coordinating mechanism) and a more recent part (involving the analyzers).

As mentioned previously, the analyzing-coordinating mechanism is composed of all those transmitting synapses with their interrelations, connected with analyzers present in the lower parts of the brain and which are directly superimposed on the corresponding sections of the coordinating mechanism, i.e., on certain groups of neurons of the reticular formation, uniting local reflex arcs along the CNS axis.

This mechanism is called upon to serve more complicated reflex coordinations connected with one or another degree of orientation in the environment. Related to them in particular are the orienting and adapting reflexes, primarily to visual and auditory stimuli (this group could also include self-adjustments of the analyzers), and reflexes which maintain the balance of the body, both static and locomotor.

In the active orientation of the organism in the external world an important part is ascribed to neurons which are especially related to processes of distribution of skeletal muscle tonus in different positions and movements of the body. The combined activity of corresponding groups of neurons, distributed at various levels of the axial part of the CNS, ensures a rapid change in the modes of tonus and tension in the muscles of the body. A similar kind of reflex coordination is also carried out with the participation of the analyzing-coordinating mechanism, attaining a particularly complex differentiation in animals with limbs possessing great freedom of movement.

Unlike the coordinating mechanism, the analyzing-coordinating formations of the brain have considerably more extensive receptor zones, located not only in adjacent, but also in remote, parts of the body and organs.

A large number of the receptors which are of major importance in carrying out the complex reflexes under discussion enter from sensory organs located in the head region, such as the retina and the cochlea of the inner ear; others are related to the equilibrium and orientation of the body in space (vestibular and otolith inner ear apparatus). This distribution causes the central transformation of corresponding impulses to be under the control of the brainstem, in which the analyzing-coordinating formations reach their highest degree of development.

In the lower vertebrates (see Figure 6) and birds there are also located the visual lobes corresponding to the superior corpora bigemina of the mesencephalon in mammals. Associated with these formations are the cerebellum, with its extensive system of bilateral connections (Figures 23 and 26), and the vestibular and other nuclei located in the brainstem and controlling the pattern of skeletal muscle tonus during the variety of positions and movements of the body. In some demersal fishes with a strongly developed sense of taste, the taste lobes of the medulla oblongata (see Figure 6), which in these animals is one of the most important parts of the analyzing-coordinating system, attain very large dimensions.

It should be noted, incidentally, that the function of maintaining the balance of the body, represented to a considerable degree in the axial part of the CNS by certain vestibular nuclei and their connections with the cerebellum and motor centers of the muscles of the eyes and the skeletal muscles of the whole body, does not develop beyond the level of the analyzing-coordinating mechanism. This apparently explains the absence of a strictly delineated representation of the vestibular system in the cerebral cortex.

There is reason to conclude that the analyzing-coordinating mechanism is represented not only in the brainstem but also in the spinal cord. The layer of transmitting neurons concentrated in the gelatinous [white] matter of the spinal cord (Figure 17) which is located at the site of entry of sensory fibers of the posterior roots into the spinal cord may also participate in this function. The white matter of the spinal cord extends directly into the white matter of the medulla oblongata and is arranged there along the pathways of sensory nuclei of some craniocerebral nerves.

The layer of neurons in the white matter is superimposed on the coordinating mechanism as an auxiliary zone of transmissions serving the afferent impulses passing in from the periphery, and farther on distributed by the reticular neurons of the gray matter of the spinal cord among the various groups of effector neurons (Figure 14). The elements under discussion are apparently adjusted to more elaborately differentiated reflex arc closures performed directly on the segmental (local) level of the spinal cord itself.

The transmissions in the white matter are of importance for the coordinating course of various local (mainly locomotor) reflexes, since they are accomplished peripherally by motor activities of multiarticular and highly mobile limbs. In mammals the neuronal fibers of the white matter, as well as neurons located higher along the analyzing-coordinating formations of the CNS, participate directly in carrying out differentiated movements of the body, conditioned by stimuli originating in the cerebral cortex.

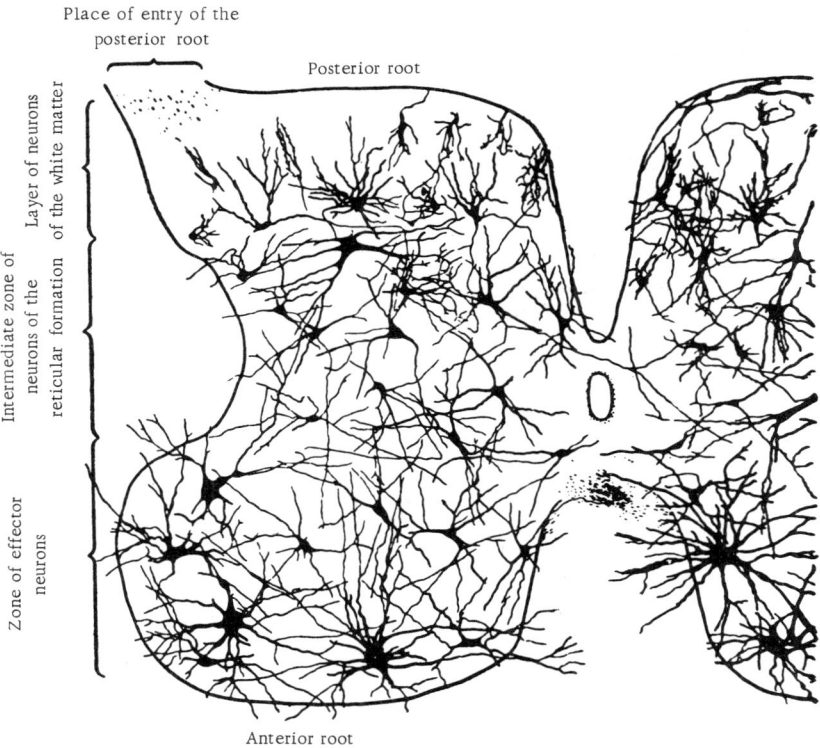

FIGURE 17. Diagram of the neuron construction of the gray substance of the spinal cord, after Zhukova. Clearly visible are the differences in detailed structure of the neurons which we relate to the analyzing-coordinating mechanism (the gelatinous matter), and which are included in the coordinating mechanism of the neurons of the reticular formation and the effector neurons (compare with Figure 30).

As indicated by Zhukova,* the white matter which functions as the integrating apparatus acting at the spinal cord level, is characterized by particular features of neuron structure which to a certain extent connect it with cortical areas (see below). The entire pattern is of a laminar type. In this zone of the gray matter of the posterior root of the spinal cord

---

* G. P. Zhukova. Nekotorye dannye v mezhneironnykh svyazyakh v spinnom i prodolgovatom mozgu (Some Data on Interneuron Connections in the Spinal Cord and Medulla Oblongata). – Arkhiv Anatomii, Gistologii i Embriologii, Vol. 39, No. 12. 1960.

(see Figure 17) the presence of a particular geometrical arrangement of neurons has been confirmed. Another characteristic feature of this zone is the presence in it of short-axon neurons or similar neurons with axons and dendritic branches. The terminal ramifications of axons of these neurons form contacts with neighboring cells, and this is typical for transmitting stations of analyzers. As Zhukova remarked later in her work, one may assume from published data that the white matter contains an organized pattern of projections of the peripheral receptors of the somatic-topical type which registers skin and kinesthetic stimuli in the regions of the corresponding segments of the spinal cord. The data mentioned above support our concept of the gelatinous matter as one of the components of the analyzing-coordinating mechanism.

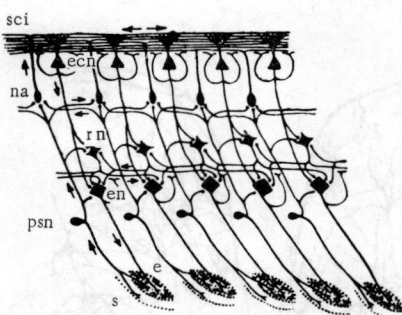

FIGURE 18. Diagram of neuronal structure of the cranial parts of analyzers forming the basic pattern in the cerebral cortex. An interconnecting network of skin- and kinesthetic analyzers is seen:

s — receptor surface of the skin; e — effector (skeletal muscle); psn — peripheral sensory neuron; en — effector neuron; nn — neuron of reticular formation; en + rn — coordinating mechanism; na — neuron included in the transmitting mechanism of the cerebral part of the analyzer, and adapted for transmission of centripetal (afferent) impulses to the cortical apparatus; ecn — efferent cortical neuron through which the centrifugal impulses are transmitted and directed to the coordinating mechanism; sci — integrated system of horizontal (tangential) connections, common to all structures of the cortical pattern type, interconnecting with efferent neurons of the cortex. This structural feature is one of the most typical aspect of the cortical pattern.

The next structural feature under discussion is the cerebral component of the analyzers, both in the axial and supraaxial parts of the CNS. This includes various zones involved in the most highly differentiated activity of the analyzing-coordinating mechanism, as well as the analyzer systems.

At all levels of the cerebral part of any analyzer, when it attains a certain degree of differentiation in carrying out analysis and synthesis of stimuli, there is a distinct multi-layer pattern (Figure 18).

Such a pattern occurs, for instance, in the taste centers of the medulla oblongata in fishes (see Figures 6 and 19A) with a strongly developed sense of taste. In animals able to perceive ultrasonic vibrations (some rodents, Carnivora, Pinnipedia), the primary auditory center of the medulla oblongata has a similar neuronal structure (Figure 19D). The cortical pattern of structure is typically present in the optic lobes (corpus bigeminum anterior of the mesencephalon (Figures 6 and 19B)) and cerebellum of all vertebrates. The cortex of the cerebellum with its particular neuron structure, as well as the cortex of the optic lobes of the mesencephalon, can be considered as a prototype of the cerebral cortex (Figure 17E).

The development of the cerebellar cortex is conditioned by the fact that the automatically functioning brain carries out analysis and synthesis of stimuli, acting on various receptor surfaces of the organism, and ensures quite complicated reflex coordinations, including the effector apparatuses of the entire body.

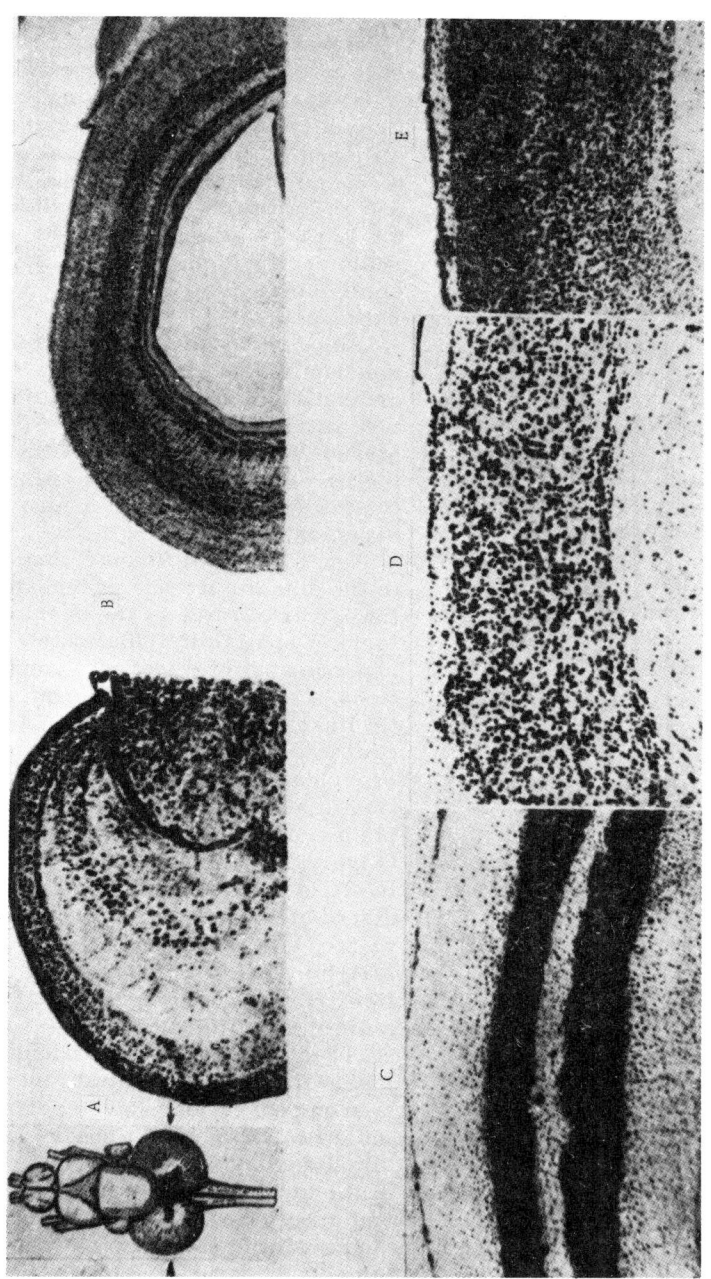

FIGURE 19. Various structural forms of the cortical laminar pattern of analyzers:

A — taste center of a fish; to the left of the microphoto is a drawing of the encephalon of a fish; the arrows point to the taste centers; B — optic lobe of the mesencephalon of a lizard; C — cortex of the cerebellum of a bird; D — auditory nucleus of the medulla oblongata of a mouse, with a structure of the cortical pattern type; E — fully developed cerebral cortex of a white rat (A, B, C, E — after V. M. Svetukhina; D — after V. P. Zvorykin).

The higher brain "terminals" of the analyzer systems, which represent the phylogenetically most recent formations of the cerebral cortex (see Figures 22 and 24), attain their highest degree of development and most complex structural differentiation of cortical patterns in some mammals. In lower vertebrates, in which the telencephalon is not yet fully developed, and devoid of cerebral hemispheres, the axial analyzing-coordinating formations already display a considerable differentiation of structure according to the cortical pattern (see Figures 6 and 19), while in the supraaxial part the latter is still represented in a rudimentary form by a primitive or semi-isolated cortex (after Filimonov).

An overgrowth of the coordinating mechanism into the analyzing-coordinating mechanism with its structure of the cortical-pattern type can already be detected in the CNS of the lower vertebrates, according to the following features of neuron organization.

The structural feature common to the spinal cord and encephalon in lower vertebrates is the special form of spatial distribution of neurons and interneuronal connections, i. e., zones of contact or synaptic links between neurons. The characteristic feature of this organization consists of a distribution in reciprocally perpendicular planes of the linked elements (Figure 20). The dendritic branches of effector and reticular neurons are distributed along the axis of the CNS mainly in a transverse direction, at a right angle to the contacting nerve fiber bundles, which are orientated mainly along the CNS axis.

These topographic relations inside the entire system of intraneuron connections have created the most favorable conditions for a simultaneous and consecutive control of the large groups of neurons included in the coordinating mechanism and propagated by central nervous conduction pathways. At the same time there is a more effective carrying out of functional possibilities inherent in the coordinating mechanism which is the main physiological task of the analyzing-coordinating mechanism. It is also evident that this type of structure represents an "apparatus of

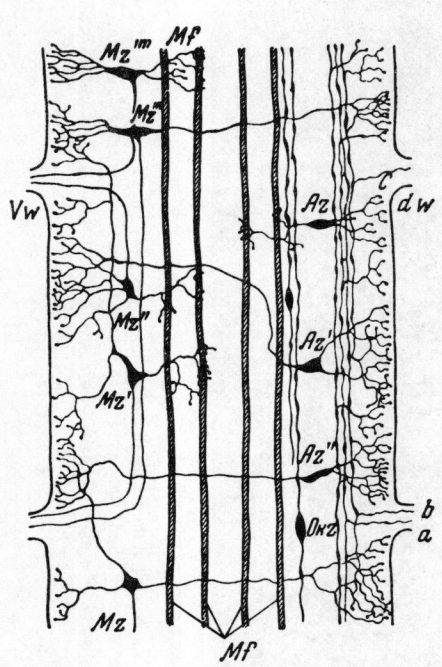

FIGURE 20. Semi-diagrammatic drawing of neuron structure of the trunk brain of a lower vertebrate (ammocoete):

a, b, c — peripheral sensory fibers entering through the posterior roots; Mz — effector (motor) neurons; Az — special transmitting neurons which we relate to the reticular formation; Mf — thick nerve fibers oriented longitudinally. To the right is presented a bundle of longitudinally oriented, thin nerve fibers constituting an extension of the fibers of the posterior roots. It can be seen that the branches of the neuronal dendrites are distributed perpendicularly to the longitudinal fibers (according to data by A. Tret'yakov from A. A. Zavarzin).

calibration" adapted to registration of strength, space, and time relations between the stimuli.

These particular structural features allow one to conclude that in lower vertebrates the coordinating mechanism along the entire axial part of the CNS reveals in a still indistinct, incompletely differentiated form, some features typical of the analyzing-coordinating mechanism.

It is most probable that this principle of organization of interneuronal connections in the CNS of the lower vertebrates forms the basis for the structure of cortical patterns seen in higher vertebrates (see Figure 18), representing the most highly organized structure of the analyzing-coordinating mechanism. The fully differentiated cortical pattern forms only a higher degree of development of neuronal-architectonic interrelations which already appear in the spinal type of vertebrate CNS.

In the evolution of vertebrates, the CNS develops as a complex formation. This involves a highly organized system of segmentary and supersegmentary reflex mechanisms, and the formation of "organizational" prerequisites for subsequent differentiation and specialization of analyzers (the analyzing-coordinating mechanism, and at a later stage, the analyzer systems), with their typical transmitting mechanisms (and the special structure of the cortical type).

5. SYSTEMS OF ANALYZERS

The consecutively linked chains of neuron transmissions which constitute the analyzer systems carry out the most complicated forms of analytic-synthetic activity of the brain which ensure a highly organized and differentiated orientation to the environment. We shall dwell briefly on the functional significance of the particular structural features which differentiate the analyzer systems from the analyzing-coordinating mechanism.

The reflex coordinations accomplished with the aid of the analyzing-coordinating mechanism are only of limited use in the combined reflex activity which serves for continuous adjustment of the organism to various special complexes of stimuli. The basic physiological purpose of this mechanism is to ensure an effective response to increasing and more complicated coordinating requirements of the organism. The analyzing-coordinating mechanism, functioning together with the coordinating mechanism, is in a position to adjust to only a limited number of stimuli, representing in a sense a neuronal association of a narrower range of action.

The formation of analyzer systems provides a means of self-determination of analyzers, and they act in the capacity of a superstructure dominating all reflex coordinations. The complex interconnections of the highest brain endings of the analyzer systems which develop extensively in vertebrate evolution (see Figure 24) reprocess the integrated data registered by all receptor surfaces of the organism. When the analyzer system differentiates further, it takes over the control of the total sum of reflex coordinations and adjusts them to function in the interest of the organism as a whole.

In the same way that the mechanisms of axial reflex coordinations are responsible for the physiologically expedient adjusting functions, one finds that in animals with separate analyzer systems the highest brain endings assume responsibility for the biological expedience of all reactions.

With the formation of analyzer systems, especially their highest brain endings, there is a qualitative change in terms of extension and a fuller ability of the organism to orient more actively to its environment; this is achieved by further improvement in the sensitivity of the physiological apparatus, involving a finer adjustment of the sense organs to perception of objects. At the same time, the organism becomes capable of counter-reacting in a more differentiated manner to the objects which stimulate it. The analyzer systems are a powerful tool, both for adjustments to conditions of the environment, and for adjustment of the environment to the requirements of the organism.

The analyzing-coordinating mechanism acts, in some way, as a "custodian" of the coordinating mechanism function introducing necessary corrections in the course of its implementation. Yet the role of the analyzing-coordinating formations is essentially limited to the further elaboration of inherent potential function in the remnants of reflex coordinations, transmitted by inheritance from ancestors. This appears especially clearly in representatives of vertebrates with an as yet incompletely developed analyzer system.

The highest brain endings of the analyzer systems in their fully developed form (formations in the fully developed new cortex together with the adjacent subcortex) possess the most complete functional possibilities to carry out more and more new "artificial" reflex coordinations throughout life, encompassing habits, skills and knowledge.

The development of the analyzer system as a single, complex interconnected formation is manifested especially in the correlation of processes of structural differentiation of the apparatuses of impulse transmission, distributed at various levels of the brain. It was noted that during intrauterine life, the separation of the cytoarchitectonic layers in the systems of visual, dermal and kinesthetic analyzers occurs at the same time as the differentiation of subcortical formations (optic thalamus and lateral geniculate body, see Figure 7) in the basic structure of nuclei (N. S. Preobrazhenskaya*, V. M. Minaeva**).

Two types of central transmitting stages, adapted to the axial and supraaxial part of the CNS, respectively, can be distinguished in the analyzer systems. Transmissions located along the axis can be related to formations of the distant subcortex, while transmissions situated in the area of transfer from the axial into the supraaxial part (optic thalami and geniculate bodies), together with subcortical nodes of the cerebral hemispheres belonging to the supraaxial part, form part of the nearest subcortex. The cortical endings of the analyzer systems are distributed within the limits of the supraaxial part (see Figures 7 and 29).

To date it may be considered a proven fact that all analyzer systems are constructed on a basis of bilateral connections between intermediate

---

* N. S. Preobrazhenskaya. Nekotorye tsitoarkhitektonicheskie dannye o razvitii korkovogo kontsa i podkorkovogo otdela zritel'nogo analizatora cheloveka (Some Cytoarchitectonic Data on the Development of the Cortical Endings and Subcortical Section of the Visual Analyzer in Man).— In: Trudy vtoroi nauchnoi konferentsii po vozrastnoi morfologii i fiziologii.—Moskva, Izdatel'stvo Akademii Pedagogicheskikh Nauk RSFSR. 1955.

** V. M. Minaeva. Stroenie korkogo kontsa i podkorkovykh obrazovanii kozhnogo analizatora v ontogeneze cheloveka (Structure of Cortical and Subcortical Formations of the Skin Analyzer in Human Ontogenesis).— Moskva, Medgiz. 1961.

and terminal links of impulse transmission chains formed by them. Those impulses are represented by corresponding peripheral, subcortical (included in the nearest and distant subcortex) and cortical areas. Each of the links is connected with the others through ascending (centripetal) and descending (centrifugal) pathways (G. L. Rasmussen,[*] S. B. Dzugaeva,[**] E. G. Shkol'nik-Yarros,[†] H. G. Kuypers and others[††]). Because of this organization of interrelations in the analyzer systems, the groups of neurons in the transmitting synapses situated between the peripheral and highest brain endings are constantly affected by the opposite flow of mutually interacting impulses. The higher brain endings of the analyzer systems are thus able to influence actively the function of neuron transmission chains participating in the transfer of centripetal impulses, stimulating some and inhibiting other groups of neurons.

The transmitting control centers of the analyzer systems included in the axial and supraaxial parts of the CNS are closely interconnected with the coordinating and analyzing-coordinating formations.

The numerous collateral branches passing out in the lower CNS levels from the analyzer systems, in the course of their ascent along the CNS axis (see Figure 7), are responsible for effecting direct contact with the corresponding sections of the coordinating and analyzing-coordinating mechanism. In this manner the analyzer systems are able, even in their axial part, to influence various reflex coordinations accomplished by the spinal cord and brainstem, by means of the interaction of centripetal and centrifugal impulses. The activities of the coordinating and analyzing-coordinating mechanisms are therefore able to alter in the same general direction in which the functional conditions of the highest brain endings of the systems of analyzers alter, following the action on them of the same centripetal afferent impulses. This mechanism ensures the timely adjustment of all reflex adaptations of the organism, accomplished along the axial part of the CNS and performed by the highest brain representations of analyzers in the supraaxial part of the CNS.

Through their connections with the reticular formation of the CNS (see Figure 7), the analyzer systems are also able to affect each other indirectly. With this the impulses entering from the analyzer systems into the reticular formation lose their specificity (modality) to some extent. The new combinations of impulses formed as a result of such interactions, through descending transmission chains of the reticular formations (the so-called non-specific activating system, see Figure 16), are able to affect the general tonus and effectiveness of function of the highest brain endings of the analyzer systems, altering their functional condition with respect to an increase or decrease in the excitability threshold.

The cortical and subcortical formations situated at the supraaxial part of the CNS have extensive bilateral connections (centripetal and centrifugal)

---

[*] G. L. Rasmussen. Further Observation on the Termination of the So-called Olivary Peduncle. — Anat. Rec., p. 106. 1950.
[**] S. B. Dzugaeva. O pryamykh svyazyakh zritel'nogo trakta s koroi golovnogo mozga (Direct Connections of the Optic Tract with the Cerebral Cortex). — Zhurnal vysshei nervnoi deyatel'nosti, Vol. 8, No. 6. 1958.
[†] E. G. Shkolnik-Yarros. Ob efferentnykh putyakh zritel'noi kory (Efferent Pathways of the Visual Cortex). — Ibid., Vol. 8, No. 1. 1958.
[††] H. G. Kuypers, A. L. Hoffman, and R. M. Beasley. Distribution of Cortical "Feedback" Fibers in the Nucleus Cuneatus and Gracilis. — "Proc. Soc. Exp. Biol. Med." p. 108. 1961.

with many groups of neurons of the axial part of the CNS (see Figures 22, 25 and 26). These connections, specialized to reinforce the counterflows of impulses, apparently form the physical apparatus for those complicated directed actions (of integration) by the higher brain endings of the analyzer systems of the total collection of reflex coordinations, and integrate them into the organism's total behavior pattern.

The development of the analyzer systems has brought about an internal reorganization of the entire neuronal structure of the coordinating and analyzing-coordinating mechanisms. This has resulted in the ability of the highest brain endings of the analyzer systems to function in a differentiated-selective manner on the effector apparatus of the body. Impulses transmitted by the supraaxial part of the CNS are capable of passing through the coordinating mechanism to the most minute groups of effector elements (the corresponding sections of the skeletal muscles of the body). With the increase in resolving ability of the analyzers, i.e., with the ever-increasing differentiation of the various stimuli registered, the organism has been able to react to them with more and more finely differentiated movements. The anatomical basis of the latter in the CNS is represented by the direct pathway of impulse transmission of neurons from the motor cortex and other cortical areas to the effector neurons of the coordinating mechanism, which are highly developed in mammals (see Figure 25). This system of centrifugal fibers connects the cortical areas of various analyzers, in particular the skin and kinesthetic ones, with the acting reflex apparatus of the axial part of the CNS. It can be considered as the pathway serving the outflow of impulse combinations, (mapped out in the cortical endings of the analyzer systems) to the effector components, as a result of an analytic-synthetic transformation of the various impulses originating from the sensory apparatus acting at the organism's periphery (see Chapter II, Section 7).

The data obtained from comparative anatomical and physiological investigations lead us to assume that in the development of the analyzer systems during vertebrate evolution, the neuron complexes included in the coordinating mechanism begin to function according to two plans; the phylogenetically older plan deals with vitally important adaptable reflex coordinations, and the phylogenetically more recent plan deals with more complex reactions carried out with the leading participation of the analyzer systems. This functional subdivision of the coordinating mechanism was fixed in the different systems of centripetal and centrifugal connections linking the neuronal groups of the corresponding CNS section with the highest brain endings of the analyzer systems.

Neuron complexes of the coordinating mechanism, formed during relatively early stages of evolution and preceding the formation of analyzer systems, retain, even in the more highly organized vertebrates, the essential function of transmitting vitally important sensory impulses to the highest brain endings of the analyzer systems. We refer here to receptor mechanisms reacting to signals originating in the internal environment of the organism, and providing vital information on multiple aspects of biological functions, and also receptors registering pain stimuli following tissue injury. All these receptor functions, accompanied by more encompassing reactions of defense and autonomic types, form a protopathic sensitivity system distinguished from the more finely differentiated, discrimination-epicritic sensitivity, associated with the function of the analyzer.

The chains of neuronal transmissions through which impulses, carrying protopathic sensitivity, reach the supraaxial parts of the CNS are localized, as determined in investigations of recent years, in certain sections of the reticular formation of the brainstem, and are intimately connected with groups of phylogenetically older nuclei of the optic thalamus present in adjacent areas of the subcortex. These formations, in turn, are linked through bilateral pathways with many areas of the cerebral cortex. This brain area possesses particularly numerous connections which are established with evolutionally older formations of the cortical pattern (primitive, old and intermediate cortex, according to I. N. Filimonov's classification), and also with those areas of the neocortex which become differentiated very early in mammalian evolution; these particular cortical centers include marginal areas of the neocortex and limbic zone, occupying the inner and lower surfaces of the cerebral hemispheres in the frontal and temporal areas (Figures 22, 46 and 47).

Because of these systems of transmission of impulses between the cerebral cortex, the reticular formations of the brainstem and midbrain ensure the integration of animal and autonomic components of reactions to vital stimuli. Further details of the physiological significance of various forms of connections between the axial and supraaxial parts of the CNS will be discussed in the next chapter.

The development of all these complex networks of transmissions during evolution, linking the axial and supraaxial CNS sections, has provided the highest cerebral cortical endings of the analyzer systems with the ability to represent in an interrelated way, and at the same time, various components of reflex activities serving different functions, adapted to other parts of the brain and the spinal cord. The constellations of neurons forming the cerebral cortex combine, according to the complicated principle of functional-topographic interdependence, various forms of interactions with the corresponding sections of the coordinating mechanism. All vertebrates have preserved chains of neuronal transmissions, adjusted to stimuli with often differentiated type, which are closely associated with protopathic perceptions in particular. In more highly developed vertebrates, such as mammals, there appear more strictly localized apparatuses of intercentral interactions, and these are adapted to the separate groups of cortical and subcortical neurons, which carry out finely adjusted and selectively directed reactions, associated with epicritic sensations.

The following observation may serve as a confirmation of this concept of functional interrelations of "specific" and "nonspecific" components in the connective systems between the cerebral cortex and lower CNS components. Animals without a cortex are incapable of carrying out local, conditioned, reflex motor acts, limited by strictly determined muscles, whereas general motor reactions, such as running to the feed box, function properly.

The complicated systemic character of functional localization in the CNS serves as a key to the understanding of the more essential aspects of its organization. Such a concept may aid in determining how the differentiation and unity of animal and autonomic functions are carried out, and how the discrimination of separate stimuli and reactions to them, along with general reactions to crude and abrupt effects on the organism from the inside, are achieved. On this basis the lower and higher levels of integration of reflex acts at various stages of differentiation are constructed, and they interrelate with the various specialized neuronal complexes.

Chapter II

REGULATION, CONTROL AND DIRECTION IN ANIMAL ORGANISMS

1. PRESENTATION OF THE PROBLEM

As far as we know, there are no precise definitions of the processes of regulation, control and direction in biological systems; these concepts are often confused or used as synonyms.

It is nevertheless obvious that the latest achievements in planning and applications of various cybernetic systems are actually based on the principle of using models of regularities occurring in living organisms. One of the most promising trends in the continuing development of cybernetics is an ever-increasing understanding of complex biological systems and the experimental reconstruction of their theoretical models. The rapid development of new disciplines such as bionomics and neurocybernetics, confirms the fact that man has increasing possibilities for creating an unlimited number of regulated, controlled and directed systems.

In view of these facts, we first attempted to formulate the concepts of regulation, control and direction in general terms — such as autoregulation, autocontrol and autodirection — and to provide specific definitions for them, based on analysis of biological objects. The factual data concerning the development of the neuronal structure of the brain in animal evolution, as described in Chapter I, were used in our elaboration of these theories. The interaction of functions described in further detail seems to encompass all manifestations of reflex activity, from the simplest to the most complicated. On the other hand, we are firmly convinced that only these concepts can explain adequately the biological and physiological significance of this activity at all stages of animal evolution.

Reflex activity is composed of processes of varying complexity and biological significance, and expresses the general regulations of development of self-organizing systems. Each type of reflex adjustment is carried out by certain morphophysiological mechanisms adapted to various CNS levels. The purpose of this and the preceding chapter is to provide a multifaceted presentation of features pertaining to the structural and functional organization of the interacting mechanisms in question.

To provide a rational explanation of reflex mechanism at different evolutionary stages, we began with the basic tenet that the well-regulated function of a system concerned with signal activity is determined by the interaction of specific components of neuronal structure and a central controller; a certain degree of local autonomy of the systems concerned is also essential. In order to elaborate our theories further, we must at this stage discuss the general problem of functional localization in the brain and follow the nature of its differentiation in the course of evolution.

2. FUNCTIONAL SIGNIFICANCE AND INTERACTIONS OF VARIOUS REFLEX MECHANISMS DIFFERING IN THEIR DEGREE OF DEVELOPMENT

Following is a description of some essential functional features of the three basic components of the neuronal system as described by us (coordinating mechanism, analyzing-coordinating mechanism and the analyzer systems), and the role they have in regulation, control and direction. We will explain these functions in relation to the three stages of progressive differentiation of the neuronal system as a whole.

In accordance with the basic theories of I. P. Pavlov, the entire reflex activity can be divided primarily into two main spheres of function, i. e., species-specific unconditioned reflexes, and individual conditioned reflex adaptations. In the course of evolution the accumulation of species experience has become fixed in reactions at varying stages of differentiation, carried out at different CNS levels, first in the spinal cord and at later evolutionary stages in the phylogenetically more recent subcortical and cortical areas of the cerebral hemispheres. These types of reaction are subordinated to relatively stable, slowly changing programming systems, formed by stages during the course of evolution of the different living species. This group of reflex adaptations, arranged in certain patterns of neuronal connections, can be isolated as an independent group of self-organizing functional systems, which we define as an "entity" composed of a collection of processes of autoregulation, autocontrol and autodirection.

The functions described above can be presented from the neurophysiological aspect in the following manner.

Autoregulation is understood by us to mean a complex of elementary animal reflex reactions of chiefly local character, and also of various autonomic reactions. Autocontrol can be defined as a complex of more differentiated animal adaptation reactions with their autonomic components, coordinating various systems of local reflexes. The function of autodirection includes the most complicated inborn (instinctive) forms of behavior, acting to serve the biological requirements of the organism. In their coordinated activation, all these functions, which may be defined as the hierarchy of unconditioned reflexes, express in their actions the various forms of species experience, and differ in their organizational level. One of the essential features of unconditioned reflex responses of different degrees of complexity, representing the accumulation of experience throughout the organism's life, is their relative independence from conditioned reflexes acquired individually by the organism. All manifestations of the latter, from the simplest to the most complicated, are concentrated in one general group of processes including regulation, control, and direction. The leading role in this group of conditioned reflex connections is referred to the direction which participates in carrying out the most complicated behavioral aspects. Control and regulation, as will be shown later on in this chapter, have an important auxiliary function in the mechanism of direction, as well as in the mechanism of autodirection. With their participation, the interaction of individual and species experience occurs, aiding in the adaptation of inborn activities of the organism to specific environmental conditions.

It may be concluded from analysis of the evolutional differentiation of brain structure, and its correlation with known experimental physiological data that the specific components of nervous activity include autoregulation, autocontrol and autodirection. Each of these components can be correlated to a certain, topographically individual, anatomical-physiological mechanism.

When autoregulation and regulation are assessed in the following discussion, these two concepts are referred to under one definition, that of autoregulation; we also use the general term autocontrol for autocontrol and control, and refer to autodirection for autodirection and direction.

The starting point of vital manifestations is undoubtedly the physiological mechanism of autoregulation, which has been responsible for the development and further elaboration of physiological adaptation mechanisms in living organisms. Plants represent, in fact, a natural autoregulating system, with adaptation possibilities limited to this function.

Animals differ from plants in their ability to perceive and adapt information on events occurring both in the outer world and in their own internal environment, and to convert them into activities serving the needs of the organism; animals possess an adequate physical organization in the form of various nerve signalization systems which are absent in plants. The quality of autoregulation inherent in all living organisms is transformed in animals into special forms of autoregulating processes, functioning through the nervous system. One of the main differences between plants and animals is the fact that in animals, reflex action is not confined only to autoregulatory processes involving signalization mechanisms. In animals more complex systems of regulation, autocontrol and autodirection have been superimposed on the more primitive mechanisms serving the basic biological needs. Thus, if plants can be characterized as autoregulating biological systems, animals represent, in addition, regulated, autocontrolled and autodirected systems which exhibit various types of "behavior." A highly organized animal organism possesses a complicated coordinated system of interconnected autoregulation, autocontrol and autodirection mechanisms.

The origin of analyzers in the animal world was conditioned mainly by the appearance of new reflex adaptations, exceeding the limits of the autoregulating biological requirements of the organism, and this determined the more and more important role of regulation, autocontrol and autodirection in the adaptation reactions of the organism. The development of these functions, and particularly of autoregulation with its most complex organization of the nervous system, was induced by the fact that in mobile organisms, with signal (impulse) activity and a good orientation in the external environment, adaptation to the latter is of increasing complexity. The animal must be able not only to store and interpret past experience, but also "anticipate" events; this contrasts with the reactions of plants, which are able to adapt only in a passive ("retrospective") way to outside changes. The active interaction of animals with the environment has of necessity led to their elaboration of more complex functions.

Autocontrol may be defined as a transitory stage between autoregulation and autodirection. It may thus be regarded also as a more primitive system preceding the more highly developed systems of autodirection and direction, at evolutionary stages at which these functions have not yet mastered autoregulation, as it occurs mainly in animals. At the autocontrol stage these functions are manifested only in individual, organized forms, and thus achieve a more complete organization of various combinations of the organism's autoregulating systems. The mechanism of autoregulation is differentiated at a very early stage in animal evolution; it is followed by autocontrol, and finally by the autodirection mechanism (see Figure 5).

A cybernetic plan as presented by A. A. Lyapunov* analyzes the differentiation in interrelationships of functions participating in the realization of various reactions of the organism at different phylogenetic and ontogenetic levels. This author considers the interaction of directing systems at various evolutionary stages as the basis of objective systemization of these functions. Biological evolution is described as a process of multiplication and selection of the directing systems. Lyapunov's interpretation of different stages of direction, apparently represents the collection of processes of autoregulation, autocontrol and autodirection, as we understand these terms.

It is assumed that the same effector apparatuses, acting as the final executive link between the reflex arcs and analyzers, serve the most diverse reflex actions, taking their course with the distinct participation of autoregulation, autocontrol and autodirection; this appears to be important, in principle, for the clarification of the basic rules of functional localization in the CNS.

The analysis and synthesis of stimuli appear to be indispensable prerequisites of a regulated reflex activity at any stage of its phylogenetic differentiation. But the processes of analysis and synthesis are manifested in different ways, depending on relations in the development of these functions. At the earliest stage of development of analyzers, represented by the analyzing-coordinating mechanism, the results of analysis and synthesis of stimuli are used in effecting autocontrol, and at a higher level of development, represented by the systems of analyzers, they are used in effecting functions pertaining to regulation, control, autodirection and direction.

Autoregulation and autocontrol (Figures 21 and 22) are related by us to reflex coordinations of the axial part of the CNS: autoregulation is related to the coordinating mechanism, autocontrol to the analyzing-coordinating mechanism. Autodirection is related to the phylogenetically older and less organized cortical sections of the higher brain endings of the analyzer systems (formations of the ancient, old and intermediate cortex (Figure 22)), together with adjacent cortical formations, i. e., the brain structures together constituting the morphophysiological basis for inborn forms of behavior (see Sections 5 and 6 of this chapter).

The higher brain endings of the analyzer systems, represented by more recent and highly organized cortical formations (formations of the fully developed neocortex; see Figures 22, 24, 46 and 47), together with the adjacent subcortex (see Figures 7 and 29), carry out, according to our concept, the most responsible function of direction. The latter is realized through effects of these sections of the higher brain endings of the analyzer

---

* A. A. Lyapunov. Ob upravlyayushchikh sistemakh zhivoi prirody i obshchem ponimanii zhiznennykh protsessov (Biological Directing Systems and the General Understanding of Vital Processes). — In: Problemy kibernetiki, Moskva, Fizmatgiz, No. 10. 1963.

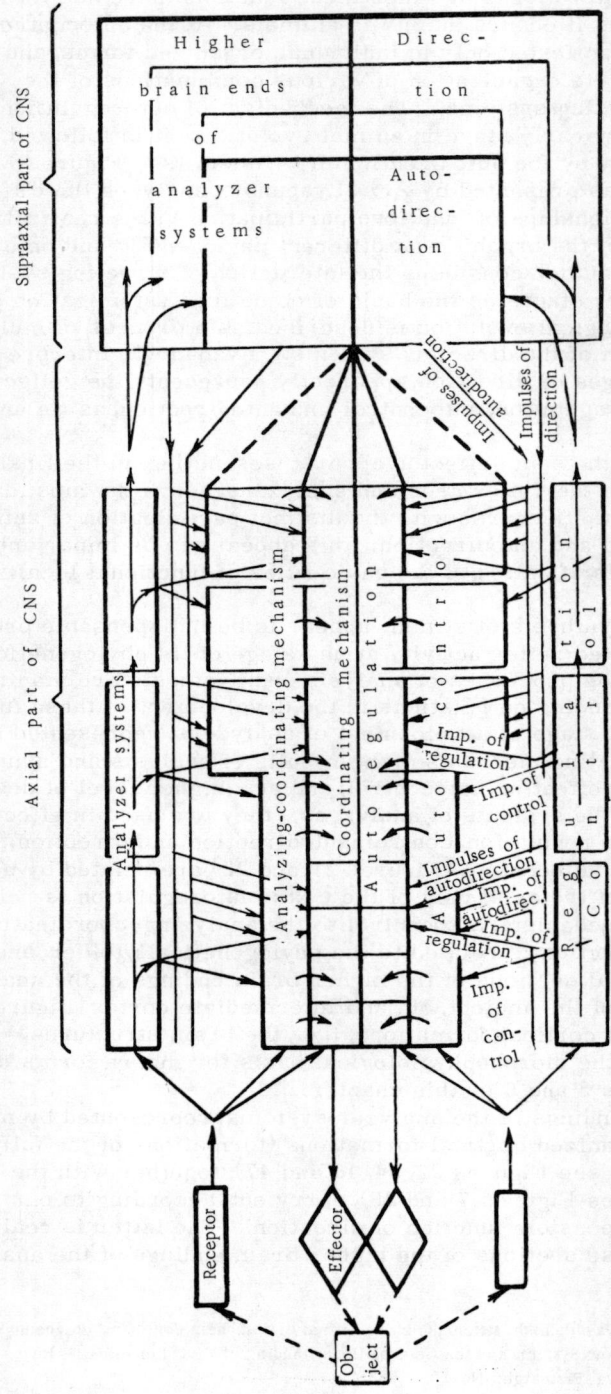

FIGURE 21. Block diagram showing relations between the various components of neuron structure (left in diagram) and functions of autoregulation, autocontrol and autodirection (right in diagram). In order to simplify the diagram, the centrifugal connections in the analyzer systems are not shown.

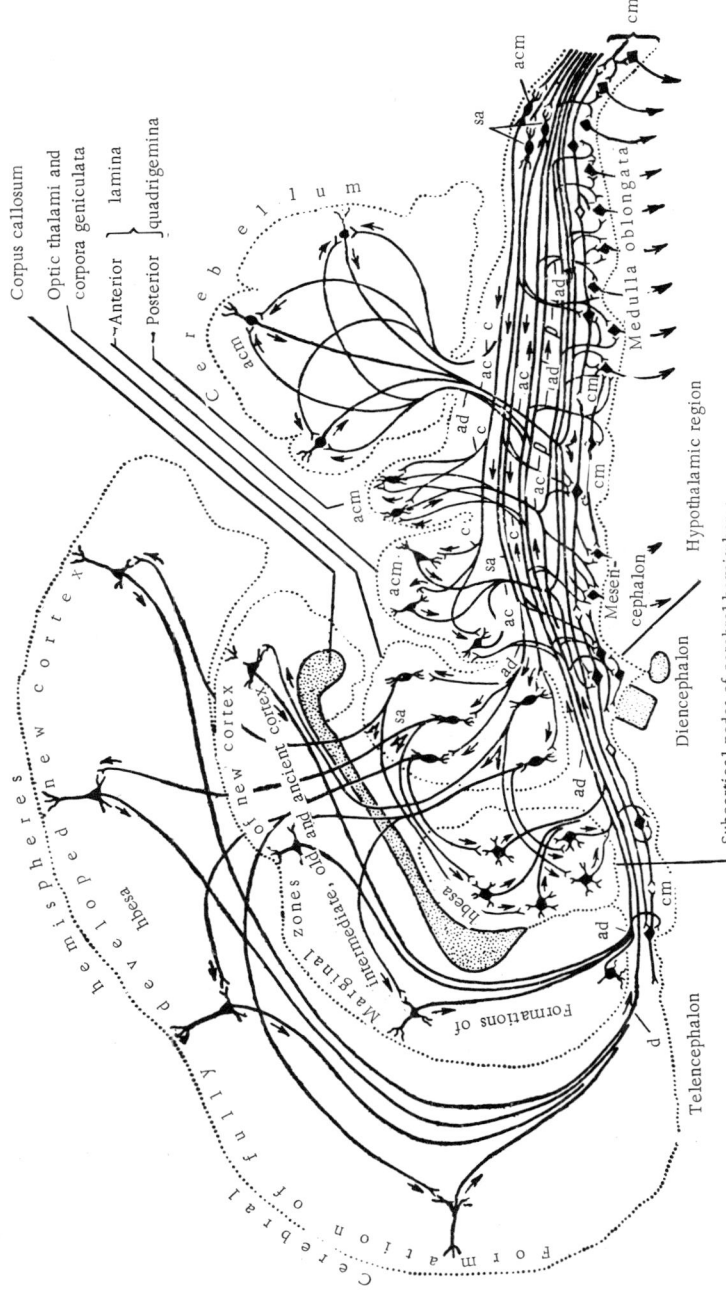

FIGURE 22. General outline of anatomical relations and connections of central nervous formations which are concerned with functions of autoregulation, autocontrol and autodirection:

hbesa — higher brain endings of analyzer systems; sa — analyzer systems; acm — analyzing-coordinating mechanism; cm — coordinating mechanism; d — impulses of direction; ad — impulses of autodirection; c — signals of control; ac — signals of autocontrol; r — signals or regulation.

systems on the older, cortical and subcortical, formations of the supraaxial part, included in the anatomicophysiological basis of autodirection, and also on mechanisms of reflex coordinations of the axial part of the CNS.

Regulation (related to the coordinating mechanism) and control (related to the analyzing-coordinating mechanism) are carried out through connections established between the coordinating and analyzing-coordinating mechanism, and the transmitting stations of the analyzer systems, localized along the axial part of the CNS (see Figures 7 and 23).

The outline of interrelations between autoregulation, autocontrol and autodirection presented above is in agreement with the concept of N. Wiener,[*] who states that the activity of the self-organizing system is based on interactions of co-subordinated algorithms at different levels. Algorithms at each of these levels ensure definite forms of reprocessing of information necessary for the realization of acts of behavior expedient for the system. The highest level is related to the production of "algorithms of self-training."

The combination of principles of relative autonomy and centralism in the activity of reflex mechanisms ensures such forms of co-subordination during which the "lower" authorities are able to carry out their special functions, and when the "higher order" components of the central nervous formations are not in control. At the same time the latter are relieved of the necessity of participating directly in the current "daily" activity of the "lower" reflex apparatuses. However, the highest CNS authorities retain the possibility of constant active intervention in the activities of the "lower" authorities, altering their control and type of response in accordance with changes in the environmental situation and other altering factors affecting behavior. We shall discuss examples of this type in the corresponding sections of this chapter.

From the short outline of functional localization, applied to the various sections of neuronal structure, it follows that reflex coordinations of the axial part of the CNS can as a whole be characterized as a complex aggregation of autoregulating and autocontrolling formations which, in their turn, are constantly affected by regulation, control, autodirection and direction. In organisms with an intact brain, the reflex coordinations of the axial part can be compared to executors responsive to impulses of autodirection together with associated impulses of regulation and control. The supraaxial part of the CNS which has achieved the highest degree of centralization (see Figure 2) has at its disposition all reflex resources of the organism, and represents the most complete tool through which the behavior of the organism as a whole is determined and directed. Behavior is planned in the highest brain endings of the analyzer systems forming this part of the CNS, and is related to the most complex types of analysis and synthesis of stimuli, based on vitally important needs of the organism. These probably reproduce adequate brain models of the outer world in the shape of images and ideas of concrete objects of satisfying requirements. These models are associated with patterns of specific functions, developed in the process of accumulation of individual experience, to be carried out when required ("motivated tasks," according to N. A. Bernshtein).

---

[*] Norbert Wiener. Cybernetics: or, Control and Communications in the Animal and the Machine. 2nd edition. — Wiley. 1961.

The continuation of the axial part of the CNS into the supraaxial part which coincides anatomically with the border between the mesencephalon and diencephalon (see Figures 2 and 7) represents the junction point of formations responsible for autoregulation and autocontrol on the one hand and autodirection on the other.

In invertebrates, autoregulation (the coordinating mechanism) seems to be related to the corporal chain of nerve ganglia (see Figure 2); autocontrol (the rudimentary analyzing-coordinating mechanism) is apparently connected with the cranial subesophageal ganglion, and the function of autodirection (rudimentary analyzer systems, specialized in these animals, mainly for fixation of species experience) is carried out by the cerebral ganglia.

The distribution and type of interaction of autoregulation, autocontrol and autodirection in complex reflex activity depend on relations in the development of the coordinating mechanism, the analyzing-coordinating mechanism and the analyzer systems. The analyzers, which represent chiefly the functions of regulation, autocontrol and autodirection, represent the physical substrate for the more complex forms of central reprocessing of impulses deriving from without and connected mainly with animal reflex actions and the relationship of the organism to the external world; only a relatively insignificant part of external impulses refers directly to the autoregulating structures of the coordinating system. On the other hand, the central reprocessing of impulses, related to the autonomic reflex action sphere, and originating from receptor surfaces sensitive to alterations in the internal environment of the organism, is linked chiefly to the coordinating mechanism and is used for processes of autoregulation of biological functions in the organism.

The principle of reciprocal connection, which is of universal significance in reflex activity of all grades of complexity, is realized in a different way in the functions of autoregulation, autocontrol and autodirection. Algorithms of reflex coordinations are fixed directly in autoregulating and autocontrolling formations of the coordinating and analyzing-coordinating mechanisms. The corresponding organization of interneuron connections (see Figures 10 and 15) ensures the function of the central apparatus of correlation and comparative evaluation of the reaction carried out with the one "programmed." Corrections in the course of actions carried out are conditioned by changes in direction of their separate components outside the borders of physiological parameters within the possibilities of the given autoregulating and autocontrolling system. According to Bernshtein,* one of the most significant conditions ensuring a coordinated course of any motivated reflex action is the supression of excess freedom of the moving organ by means of sensory corrections. This allows for the movement to acquire a dynamic stable form, i.e., it becomes an autoregulated, autocontrolled and autodirected process.

The central apparatuses of comparison of the final result of the reaction with the originally planned "program" are localized along all levels of the CNS. The components which have the highest authority in this activity are connected with those components of neuronal structure which carry out the functions of autodirection and direction. Bernshtein's studies on motivated

---

* N. A. Bernshtein. Ocherednye problemy fiziologii aktivnosti.(Future Problems of the Physiology of Activity).— In: Problemy kibernetiki, No. 6, Moskva, Fizmatgiz. 1961.

coordinations have convincingly demonstrated that the necessary corrections in the process of effecting the consecutive stages of functions under question are introduced by the transmitting formations of the analyzer systems distributed along the different CNS levels. In this manner afferent syntheses and the recoding of transmitted impulses are set in specific patterns, which direct the course of corresponding components of the integral motivated act.

3. AUTOREGULATION AND REGULATION

As already mentioned in Chapter I, Section 3, the autoregulating structures are correlated in action with physiological processes which are more elementary and older phylogenetically and ontogenetically, and which aid in maintaining a stable uniformity of reflex adaptations developed during the evolution of a given animal species. Along with autoregulations of various biological functions in the animal organism by means of the autonomic nervous system (see Figure 12), one must include various components of static and locomotor reflexes, as well as other elementary, defense, adaptational and nutritional reflexes. All autoregulations of this category are known to be involuntary, unconscious reflex functions. In the anatomical-physiological arrangement they are subject to the control of local segmental reflex arcs which, together with the suprasegmental apparatus that unites them, are included in the coordinated mechanism.

Any reflex coordination related to the coordinating mechanism represents, in our view, a definite autoregulating structure, formed from the experience of many generations. The coordinating mechanism as a whole, with its segmentary and suprasegmentary sections, represents the anatomical-physiological basis for the evolutionary earliest autoregulating reflex adaptations of the organism.

All local segmentary reflexes are known to function according to the principle of a linked functional agonist-antagonist pair (see Figure 10). The agonistic and antagonistic components can thus be considered as two linked members of an elementary biological autoregulating system. The distinct structural features of the latter ensures the automatic rectifying of deviations of the system from normal physiological standards. It is precisely the principle of reciprocal innervation which originates and appears at the time of establishment of the animal's autoregulating system, that is, as stated, the basis of regulated reflex activity.

Taking into consideration the investigations of L. A. Orbeli[*] concerning the role of the cerebellum in the adaptive-trophic processes associated with the sympathetic nervous system, it may be assumed that some autonomic autoregulations are carried out with some participation of autocontrol, i. e., they depend on the analyzing-coordinating mechanism. Regulation, as opposed to autoregulation, refers to a physiological mechanism related to the axial parts of the analyzer systems. It is concerned with control of the autoregulating adaptive functions carried out by the coordinating mechanism

---

[*] L. A. Orbeli. Izbrannye Trudy. T. 2. Adaptatsionno-troficheskaya funktsiya nervnoi sistemy (Selected works. Vol. 2. Adaptive-Trophic Function of the Central Nervous System). — Moskva-Leningrad, Izdatel'stvo AN SSSR. 1962.

intimately related to various reflex activities which are determined by the general orientation of the organism to its environment. Physiologically these responses are associated with the analyzer systems and their connections with the coordinating mechanism.

One of the morphological components related to the function of regulation consists of the numerous collateral branchings, proceeding along the axial part of the CNS to the segmentary and suprasegmentary formations of the coordinating mechanism, and arising from the transmitting ganglia and bundles of centripetal fibers included in the analyzer systems (see Figure 7). The collateral branchings under discussion are directed simultaneously to the reticular formation and to the effector (motor) neurons of the spinal cord and the brainstem.

Through these interneuronal connections the currents of impulses proceeding into the higher (supraaxial) brain endings of the analyzer systems, and transformed into impulses of autodirection, are able to act simultaneously on the total autoregulating physiological system of the organism. Since the neurons included in the transmitting ganglia located in the axial parts of the analyzers and connected with the coordinating mechanism are constantly influenced by centripetal and centrifugal impulses, the latter are able to change the condition of the coordinating mechanism in different directions. Additional forces for the rapid mobilization of all reflex actions of the organism are thus set free, and are able to function in accordance with given external stimuli affecting the biological equilibrium of the organism.

It seems that the less developed the analyzer systems in animals are, the less pronounced is their regulating effect on the activity of the coordinating mechanism and the more pronounced are the "free" reactions, i.e., those not subjected to autodirection or autoregulation (see Section 9 of this chapter).

These statements aid in clarifying the importance of auxiliary regulation in the functions of autodirection.

4. AUTOCONTROL AND CONTROL

The basic physiological purpose of autocontrol is to ensure complex interactions between various autoregulations of the organism in conformity with its active orientation in the external environment. This function finds its "organizational-morphological" expression in the analyzing-coordinating mechanism. In comparison with the coordinating mechanism, this mechanism encompasses more intricate complexes of autoregulating systems, and leads the adaptive potentialities of the organism to conform to a wider range of changes in the external environment.

Reflex coordinations connected with the analyzing-coordinating mechanism represent complex associations of autoregulating adaptations, mainly in animals. "Inspection" is necessary for their regulated course and autocontrol appears exactly in that role. These reflex coordinations (taking their course automatically and involuntarily) can be defined as autocontrolling autoregulations.

Qualitative differentiation of autocontrolling apparatuses from the simple autoregulating ones consists of the following.

Autoregulating mechanisms are concerned with a relatively narrow range of physiological parameters, rigidly determining the regime of their activity, and not exceeding those conditions which are directly connected with the type of activity taking place. In contrast, the autocontrolling structures, representing an already more or less complex physiological aggregate of autoregulating systems, function with a certain calculation of changes taking place outside the direct sphere of application of stimuli, acting on various autoregulating systems included in this setup.

Autocontrol activity unites various reflexes which maintain body equilibrium, as well as static and locomotor reflexes, carried out with participation of the vestibular apparatus, cerebellum, visual analyzer, and receptors present in all skeletal muscles and skin. The same category of reflex coordinations, taking their course with participation of autocontrol, include various orienting reflexes, acting by means of the lower brain components of the analyzers, as well as adaptation reflexes of a certain degree of differentiation and reflexes of self-adjustment of analyzers to the action of stimuli (for instance, the interaction of different forms of muscle tonus, change in diameter of the pupil in accommodation and convergence, etc.).

The cerebellum, with its highly developed complexity of connections (Figure 23), and with the transmitting ganglia in the brainstem under cerebellar control, may be likened to a highly effective controlling structure, ensuring the normal course of various reflex coordinations but affecting the body as a whole. This automatically and unconsciously functioning "superior organ" of autocontrol integrates the activity of several physiological systems: skeletal muscles, the organ of equilibrium (vestibular and otolithic apparatuses), visual receptors; it also coordinates the systems to function as a response to autodirection, originating from the highest brain endings of the analyzer system (see Figure 26).

In lower vertebrates (see Figure 6) the optic lobes are also an important correlating center which aid in carrying out complex coordinations of motor function, on the basis of a functional association set in action by various sense organs.

The reflex adaptations produced during the life of the entire species are the main area of application of autocontrol and autoregulation. In this case, however, autocontrol depends to a greater extent on the function of autodirection than on the processes of autoregulation. We came to this conclusion because the more complex inborn reflex adaptations (e.g., static and locomotor) performed with the participation of the cerebellum, not only in man but also in many animals, require initial training. In this type of anatomical-physiological correlations there is a close functional interconnection between the lower and higher brain components of the analyzers.

The physiological mechanism of autocontrol, like the mechanism of autoregulation, has a high degree of autonomy in relation to the higher brain control centers. Evidence of the relative functional independence of both the autocontrolling and the autoregulating structure of analyzer systems, and especially those of the higher supraaxial sections, is provided by the following facts.

A decerebrated cat can perform a series of complex motor reflex coordinations in running, jumping, even climbing trees. At the same time, in such an animal devoid of the cerebral hemispheres all biological direction

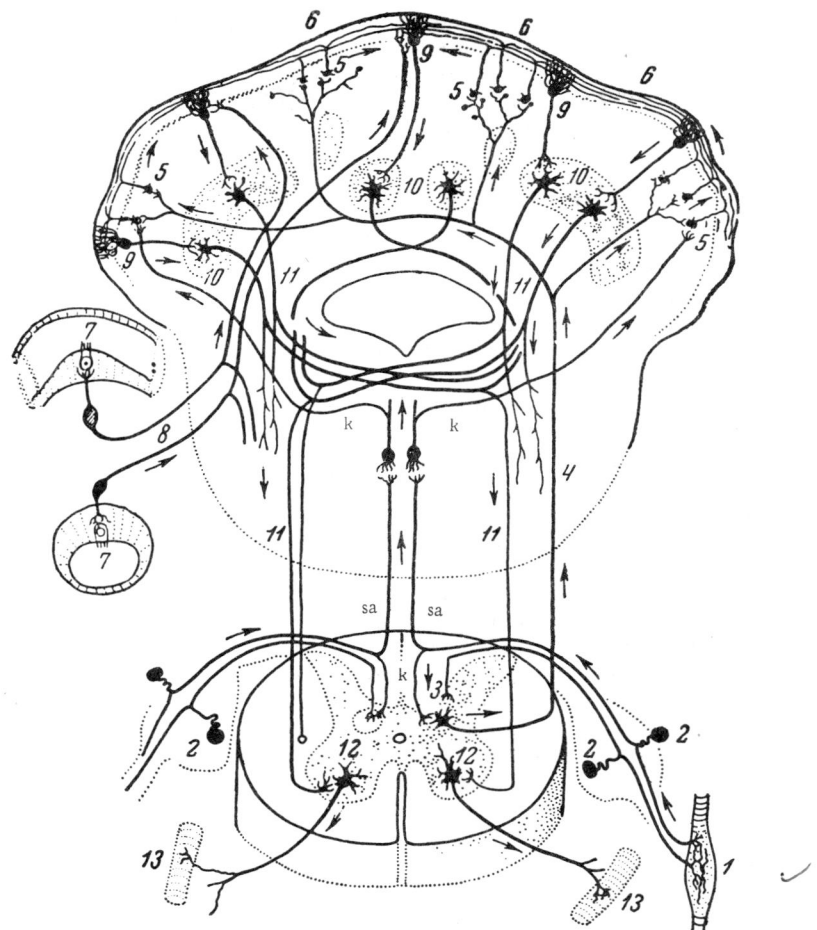

FIGURE 23. Outline of neuronal transmissions and cerebellar connections:

1 — receptor ending of a sensory neuron fiber in a skeletal muscle; 2 — peripheral sensory neuron in a ganglion; 3 — transmitting neuron in the spinal cord projected in the cerebellum; 4 — centripetal pathways from the spinal cord into the cerebellum; 5 — transmitting elements (cells — ganglia) in the cerebellar cortex; 6 — horizontal bundles produced by fibers of these neurons, establishing contact with efferent neurons of the cerebellar cortex — Purkinje's cells (9); 7 — receptors of the orthostatic organ (vestibular and otolithic apparatuses of the inner ear); 8 — centripetal pathways from the orthostatic organ to the cerebellum; 9 — efferent neurons of the cerebellar cortex (Purkinje's cells) sending impulses referred by the reflex centers of skeletal muscles; 10 — transmitting nuclei on the pathways of transmission of these impulses, located under the cerebellar cortex; 11 — pathways of the centrifugal impulses from the cerebellum to the spinal cord; 12 — effector neuron of the spinal cord innervating a skeletal muscle; 13 — motor nerve ending in voluntary (skeletal) muscle; sa — analyzer systems; k — offshoots of the analyzer systems into the transmitting ganglia, included in the connections of the cerebellum (after Cajal, with some additions).

is lost because of a lack of impulses referable to autodirection. The animal is incapable of altering its behavior in a guided manner, i.e., to ensure adequacy of conditions and activities of the organism in situations due to environmental changes. Such animals become actual "living reflex automatons," preserving the ability to carry out even relatively complex coordinations, but losing the capacity to sense and react to "intelligent" information.

An animal in which the most frontally located (supraaxial) parts of the cerebrum are removed acts to some extent as a "marionette" which only moves when its string is pulled. Reflex responses induced by corresponding stimuli, although fully regulated, are not integrated to a whole and do not constitute "behavior."

We determine the difference between autocontrol and control on the basis of the same anatomical-physiological principles as between autoregulation and regulation.

As already stated, we consider the physiological control system directing the activity of the autocontrolling mechanisms an important link in individual adaptation. It acts through the axial sections of the analyzer systems; some of its morphological components are the connections established in the course of evolution between the lowest (spinal cord and brainstem) transmitting neuronal elements of the analyzer systems and the analyzing-coordinating formations, distributed along the CNS axis (Figure 23k). The flow of impulses distributed in the transmitting ganglia of the analyzer systems and the functional condition of the analyzing-coordinating mechanism change through impulses carried by the connections mentioned before, in conformity with the changes occurring under the influence of the same impulses in the higher brain endings of the analyzer systems. Since the analyzer systems include, in addition to pathways of centripetal impulses, pathways leading impulses in a centrifugal direction as well, the mechanisms of regulation and control, in their direction of autoregulating and autocontrolling mechanisms, are able to account not only for the type of stimuli, but also for various states of the higher sections of the brain.

The type of reactions carried out, their directions, duration and intensity, determine the impulses of regulation and control, distributed along the axial parts of the CNS, and determine the shift in activity of the corresponding autoregulating and autocontrolling systems of the organism from one level to another. These functional shifts actually act in the capacity of auxiliary functions which are applied by the regulation mechanisms to carry out the commands of autodirection originating in the highest CNS components. These commands cannot be fully carried out without the intervention and auxiliary action of regulation and control.

5. GENERAL CHARACTERISTICS OF AUTODIRECTION AND DIRECTION

Autodirection and direction can be described as two closely interconnected functions of parts of the brain of a single origin. These functions are significant for the organism because the constructive possibilities of the autoregulating and autocontrolling apparatuses are in themselves inadequate for the solution of complex tasks arising in more highly developed animals in the process both of their active daily adaptation to environmental changes, and of external changes and their effects on their needs. These processes depend primarily on determining the effects of various biological factors on the organism, and the expedient use of reactions, including those inherited or acquired. Thus, all autoregulating and autocontrolling reflex adaptations of which a certain organism is capable result from its general orientation in the environment, and from evaluating the significance of events affecting it.

Autodirection and direction in contrast to autoregulation and autocontrol represent a more complex and differentiated type of reflex activity. The anatomical representations of these functions are found in the higher cerebral endings of the analyzer systems; their origin is in the telencephalon, and they develop progressively during vertebrate evolution. The formations of the higher cerebral endings are represented in the highly developed vertebrates by the cerebral hemispheres with their cortical and subcortical formations (see Figure 22). They are of decisive importance in the integration of the entire range of behavior, physiologically representing the organ responsible for higher nervous activity, in accordance with Pavlov's definition.

According to the investigations by E. A. Asratyan, E. Sh. Airapet'yants* and others, the cerebral cortex is the most active center in the organization of defense-adaptive activities, directed to the compensation of disturbed functions referable to the lower CNS areas. Cortical control ensures well-functioning reflex coordinations which compensate for any defects in the system of newly developed conditioned reflex connections. New coordinations are thus formed to replace the ones which have ceased to function. In animals lacking a cortex the range of adaptive and compensatory activities is severely restricted.

Since the higher cerebral endings of the analyzer systems are related to the most complex forms of analysis and synthesis of stimuli, and ensure the most competent orientation in the external world, they represent a highly perfected instrument which allows the organism to foresee events and direct its activities accordingly, on the basis of past experience. These complex formations of the telencephalon are the true controllers of the sum total of the organism's behavior, i. e., they represent the most important development of higher nervous activity monitoring the functions of direction in its broadest aspect, autodirection. In accordance with the definition by U. R. Eshbi,** the ability to reason eventually forms the various aspects of the processes of direction.

The mechanism of autodirection, centered in the brain and used in the formation of strategic forms of behavior, carries out the selection and programming of the reactions, actions and operations accomplished in a definite consecutive order. "Refusal" of the function of autodirection appears, most characteristically, precisely in those cases in which the

---

* E.Sh. Airapet'yants. Opyt sravnitel'nogo izucheniya printsipa zameshchaemosti v mezhanalizatornoi integratsii (Experimental Comparative Study of the Principle of Substitution and Inter-Analyzer Integration). — In: Voprosy sravnitel'noi fiziologii analizatorov. Izdatel'stvo LGU. 1960.

** U. R. Eshbi. Chto takoe razumnaya mashina (What is a Reasoning Machine). — In: Vozmozhnoe i nevozmozhnoe v kibernetike, Moskva, Izdatel'stvo AN SSSR. 1963.

function of selection of one particular solution for a given problem, from several alternatives, cannot be realized for various reasons. As U.R. Eshbi remarks, under such conditions "a misplaced type of behavior" is not seldom noted. Thus, for instance, when two opposing stimuli act on a chaffinch, such as fear of the feed box and the wish to get to the food, the bird may behave strangely by beginning to clean its feathers with its beak, etc.

Autodirection represents the final highly developed stage of analytic-synthetic transformation of the entire signalling system reaching the higher cerebral endings of the analyzer systems from outside as well as from inside the organism. In this sequence of processes we see the natural expression of the necessary prerequisite for the general principles governing reception of comprehensive information during all environmental conditions, in any organized system capable of realization of the function of autodirection.

Autodirection may in fact be defined as the ability of the organism, in accordance with external situations, to accept or encourage some and exclude or reduce other reflex coordinations and perform various commutations from one coordination to another, as well as change the direction of their function and the type of their interactions.

The significance of autodirection systems increases progressively in animal phylogenesis. They become much more complex and differentiated as they gain more and more specialized functions of autoregulation and autocontrol. This pattern may be demonstrated, for instance, by the fact that in the more highly organized invertebrate representatives (crustaceans and insects), extirpation of the brain results in a greater degree of defective orientation in the environment, and more pronounced disorders in behavior than in the lower and less organized animal forms (worms). Differences in reactions to stimuli and in autodirection are even more obvious in vertebrates, depending on the organizational level of their higher nervous centers in the brain.

Interaction and interrelation of functions of autodirection are generally determined by the total aggregation of components of behavior, both inborn and acquired during life, which characterize each animal species.

6. AUTODIRECTION ("RESTRICTED," OR AUTOMATIC DIRECTION)

The term autodirection, which can also be defined as "restricted," or automatic direction, and which represents the phylogenetically older stage of development of the mechanisms of control, implies the presence of forms and components of behavior which have been fixed during evolution as complex chains of inborn adaptive reactions, of vital importance for the organism and the entire species (vital reactions). These include all instinctive forms of behavior, the programs of which have been fixed as a result of experience of former generations during centuries and are transmitted as factors inherited from parents to their progeny. In man, such reactions are largely involuntary.

Autodirection appears most clearly as a basic behavior pattern in some of the higher invertebrates (for instance, insects). The automatisms of observed behavior in insects are so perfected, "polished" through the process of natural selection, that they create the impression of pseudo-reasoning ability. Some vertebrates, such as fish and birds, use such automatisms, collected during the history of development of the species, for adaptation to the environment, with great effectiveness.

The anatomical structures involved in autodirection in vertebrates are, as already mentioned, the phylogenetically older formations of the higher brain centers (see Figure 22). The latter include the formations of the old, or semi-isolated cortex and the more primitive sections of the isolated cortex (old cortex or hippocampus, and intermediate cortex, according to the classification of I. N. Filimonov),* together with sections of the sub-cortical basal ganglia in the cerebral hemispheres and diencephalon connected with these formations (complex of the amygdaloid nucleus, the phylogenetically old nuclei of the optic thalamus and nuclei of the hypo-thalamic region). In higher vertebrates (mammals), some formations of the new cortex of lower functional significance may also be considered as part of the brain substrate of autodirection. We refer to the marginal zones of the new cortex (see Figures 46 and 47): the limbic and insular zones, together with formations of the so-called mediobasal cortex (certain parts of the frontal and temporal cortex on the inner and lower surfaces of the cerebral hemispheres). These sections of the brain are directly related to the morphological-physiological mechanisms of vital reactions and emotional behavior, as has been shown in recent experiments (K. Pribram).**

The patterns of instinctive forms of behavior vary widely in different vertebrate representatives of different levels of development; there is a correlated difference in the morphological-physiological basis of the function of autodirection in different animals. It is interesting to note that from the point of view of structural and functional uniformity, precisely in those vertebrates whose behavior is determined by autodirection the higher brain formations are specialized mainly for hereditary fixation of species experience. In fish the relatively little developed higher brain formations (see Figure 6) are represented by the oldest formation of the semi-isolated cortex; in birds almost the entire cerebral hemispheres are formed from hypertrophied subcortical ganglia, while the cortical formations have become significantly reduced, even as compared with those in reptiles.

7. DIRECTION PROPER ("FREE," OR VOLUNTARY, AND AUTOMATIZED (AUTOMATIC))

The broad range of activity of the direction mechanism can be sub-divided into two types:

---

* I. N. Filimonov. Sravnitel'naya anatomiya kory bol'shogo mozga mlekopitayushchikh. Paleokorteks, arkhikorteks i mezhutochnaya kora (Comparative Anatomy of the Mammalian Cerebral Cortex. Paleocortex, Archicortex and Intermediate Cortex). — Moskva, Izdatel'stvo AMN SSSR. 1949.

** K. Pribram. K teorii fiziologicheskoi psikhologii (Theory of Physiological Psychology). — Voprosy Psikhologii, No. 2. 1961.
K. Pribram. Perspektivy razvitiya neiropsikhologii (Prospects of Development of Neuropsychology). — Voprosy Psikhologii, No. 2. 1964.

a) "free" or voluntary (in man, conscious) direction;
b) automatized (realized unconsciously in man) direction.

As "free" we define the type of behavior which is conditioned by the total aggregation of changes in the environment, both those happening at a given moment and those assimilated from past experience. The prerequisite of such behavior based on complex systems of conditioned reflex connections is the ability of the organism to become orientated in those qualities of the environment which characterize its "personal," individual life. Such patterns of behavior are determined by inborn reaction only in their general tendency. Voluntary, "free" behavior differs most significantly from "restricted" automatic behavior because it is formed individually on the basis of training and accumulation of experience during life. The sum of both "natural" reflex coordinations, inherited by the given organism from its ancestors, and "artificial" ones, those formed during life, is available for the basic task of adaptation to individual conditions of existence thanks to voluntary direction. Thus, this type of direction is manifested by patterns of behavior which are referable to a unified activity of analysis and synthesis of stimuli and conditioned reflex completion.

It must be emphasized that the concept of "voluntary" direction includes various forms of behavior such as "voluntary" behavior in animals (Pavlov) and specific human active conscious activity, expressed in speech.

J. M. Sechenov defined as "voluntary" those movements which are directed with a definite conscious aim, and which are themselves objects of consciousness. Pavlov included in his concept of voluntary activity the most highly developed analysis and synthesis of impulses proceeding on the level of the cerebral cortex and providing continuous information on each activity. In accordance with the theories of a number of Soviet psychologists (L. S. Vygodskii,* A. N. Leont'ev,** A. V. Zaporozhets† and others) in man the voluntary actions are directed by the image of the final result, and are formed with the participation of the second signalling system. I. S. Beritov†† also considers all behavioral reactions conditioned by reproduction of models (images) of external objects in the cerebral cortex as voluntary. He defines voluntary action involving manipulation of objects as "instrumental actions."

Voluntary direction is thus the final result of an analytic-synthetic transformation of the entire signalization complex perceived by the sense organs and transmitted to the highest cerebral (cortical) endings of the analyzer systems.

According to U. R. Eshbi's definition, the function of direction can also be represented as an activity of "the reasoning system" which is capable of performing a suitable selection on the basis of effective reprocessing of received information. Eshbi relates man's ability to reason to the

---

* L. S. Vygodskii. Razvitie vysshikh psikhicheskikh funktsii (Development of the Highly Evolved Mental Functions). — Moskva, Izdatel'stvo APN RSFSR. 1960.

** A. N. Leont'ev. Problemy razvitiya psikhiki (Problems of Development of the Mind). — Moskva, APN RSFSR. 1959.

† A. V. Zaporozhets. Razvitie proizvol'nykh dvizhenii (Development of Voluntary Movements). — Moskva, Izdatel'stvo APN RSFSR. 1960.

†† I. S. Beritov. Nervnye mekhanizmy povedeniya vysshikh pozvonochnykh zhivotnykh (Nervous Mechanism of Behavior in Higher Vertebrates). — Moskva, Izdatel'stvo AN SSSR. 1961.

mechanisms of human direction. In human society, educational and training processes which assist the direction of formation and development of mental activities and individual personality traits are manifested in one of the oldest and most important forms of directed action, e.g., directions in the sphere of interhuman relations.

A. I. Berg* defines direction as a process of transferring a complex dynamic system from one state to another through action on its variables.

In the complex process of direction in both living organisms and machines, V. A. Trapeznikov** differentiates three main functional groups: study of the directed object, development of the strategy and tactics of direction, realization of the strategy and tactics of direction. The organism as a whole is seen as a system of optimal direction.

N. A. Bernshtein's concept is of significant value in understanding the role of direction in the formation of active behavior. This concept is based on the assumption that behavior is conditioned by a situation, but is not fully determined by it. The organism is confronted with the necessity of deciding on a definite mode of action, represented as a model of a "necessary future," "coded" in the brain.

According to Bernshtein, the solution of a task requiring action consists of the following two main factors:

a) probable prognosis of a future situation based on current information perceived, i.e., extrapolation of changes in the situation during a certain period of time to come;

b) programming of action expected to lead to attainment of the target action.

Such programming of action represents an interpolation of the situation in question and the one considered "necessary" for the individual. It follows that the organism does not simply react to a situation or to a signal-significant stimulus initiated by it; it is confronted with the necessity of taking into account the dynamics of its changes and implementing a probable prognosis and, following that, selecting a method of behavior. Evaluation of a future situation with no more than some degree of probability and active selection of action in response to the situation, not conditioned by its directing signal — this, according to Bernshtein, to a great extent distinguishes the active behavior of a living organism from that of a reacting machine of any degree of precision or complexity.

We assume that this mechanism of comparative evaluation of a given situation with a desirable one, and the interpolation and selection of activity represents the typical difference between behavior of higher animals (depending on the function of the direction proper) from that of lower animals, in whom this function is still poorly developed or absent. It is typical that the behavior of more primitive in contrast to more highly developed animals is not only conditioned by the situation on hand, but is either partially or fully determined by it (see Section 9 of this chapter). In other words, the more primitive animal can estimate a probable prognosis of the future and program its behavior accordingly, but to a very limited degree.

---

* A. I. Berg. Kibernetiku na sluzhbu kommunizmu (Cybernetics in the Service of Communism). — In: "Vozmozhnoe i nevozmozhnoe v kibernetike." Moskva, Izdatel'stvo AN SSSR. 1963.

** V. A. Trapeznikov. Kibernetika i avtomaticheskoe upravlenie (Cybernetics and Automatic Direction). — In: "Vozmozhnoe i nevozmozhnoe v kibernetike." Moskva, Izdatel'stvo AN SSSR. 1963.

Automatic direction is based on consecutively interconnected formulae of motor coordinations, formed "artificially" during life; reflex formations present at birth, are used in conjunction as "raw" material.

In analyzing the automatic pattern of voluntary movements and activity associated with their transformation into involuntary ones, it would be advisable to refer to Bernshtein's comprehensive theory of coordinating levels of the CNS and the correlated "transciphered" ("transcoded") series of impulses in the process of their transmission from various coordinating levels to others.

Bernshtein postulates that the development of a habit is not simply the mastering of various motor acts by means of repetition, but a process of constant perfection of a certain motor pattern, e.g., the active search for more and more adequate, optimal and rational variations of problem solving (in the form of trials and attempts to select suitable responses, etc., in the pre-automatic period).

According to Bernshtein's* definition, automatism represents a process of staged transmissions of "background" components of the motor act to the levels of corresponding corrections, accomplished by adequate, selective syntheses, and of structures in "programming" responses. An example of such a correcting transmission associated with automatization of a movement is provided by the transfer of performed functions from the state of spatial perception to the state of defining the outline of the body of the organism concerned; the assimilated motor habit is subsequently carried out without the participation of visual control. Various transfers of training are also possible ("exercises in habit"), i.e., the use of automatic actions previously developed for another habit (e.g., riding a bicycle, skating) for construction of a new habit of automatic acts. According to Bernshtein locomotion is also included in the ready background components already assimilated during the early period of development and used later for the formation of new habits and experiences.

The fuller and more reliably a motor habit is assimilated, the richer is the background of "coordinating resources," and the broader is the range of variants and complications of the task in which the attained degree of automatism is maintained. This aids in maintaining a wide range of all components of acquired and adaptable variations of the organism's functions.

Stabilization of a habit implies the degree of its resistance to adverse influences (interferences) caused by its de-automation. The final stage of the process of automation is conditioned by activation of the entire aggregate of background levels and standardization of the habit according to its motor composition. Standardization of a habit is connected with ensuring the exchange of fixation of efforts to maintain tension of the corresponding synergistic muscles, limiting movement of the part of the body by the previously fixed route. A significant role in this process is ascribed to the flexible physiological mechanism which enables the organism to apply the various reactive and inertial forces emerging during realization of the movement and use them for correction at later periods.

I. S. Beritov defines the processes of automatism as chains of conditioned reflexes by means of which voluntary acts become fixed in continuing

---

* N. A. Bernshtein. O postroenii dvizhenii (Construction of Movement). — Moskva, Medgiz. 1947.

repetition under similar conditions. Such automatic involuntary behavior ceases as soon as the usual conditions change; the behavior of the animal then begins to be determined by active orientation in the environment, and this is expressed in active selection of actions directed by images of corresponding subjects.

The acquired motor coordinations, formed primarily as a result of repeated stimuli originating in voluntary direction, acquire an involuntary "machine type" character only as a secondary effect, as a result of exercise and training, and take their course in man without the permanent and active participation of consciousness. These types of processes are the underlying factors in the formation of various habits (professional, athletic, etc.). The more complex automatic acts composed of a series of motor coordinations include the behavior of a person under hypnosis (see next section of this chapter). An example of fully automatic forms of behavior occurring without the participation of voluntary direction is provided by the actions of a somnambulist walking along the cornice of a building.

The category of automatized direction also includes the most complex intracortical "mental coordinations" supported by the combined activity of corresponding groups of neurons which represent the physical basis for the intellectual activities taking place in the cerebral cortex. We are referring to the so-called "mental activities" (P. Ya. Gal'perin[*]) which originally, in their process of development in a child, take their course as actual manipulation of objects ("materialized actions") with the constant participation of consciousness. Later these functions are converted from external to internal ones (become "interiorized"), setting a definite pattern needing no further constant voluntary direction.

It follows from our concept of automatic processes that there is a principal difference between automatic direction and inborn automatisms of behavior which characterize autodirection and which are fully predetermined by biological tendencies specific to any species as a whole.

A clear distinction must be made physiologically between "automatic" and "automatized" processes in the animal organism, although both these types of manifestation are related to the sphere of involuntary reflex activities of the organism. The first, in contrast to the second, require no preliminary training, since the organism is born with ready formulae determining the course of corresponding reactions. To a greater or lesser degree, this principle of reflex automatic function determines all autoregulating and autocontrolling systems of the axial part of the CNS; as mentioned, the same principle also determines autodirection.

Any conditioned reflex reaction formed with the participation of voluntary direction (new "artificial" motor or secretory coordination) may also be regarded with respect to the mechanism of its origin as an expression of a particular "automatism"; the one difference is that in these cases those components of the completed process which are not contained in the total experience of the entire species are subjected to automatization. In contrast, the forms of behavior manifested as a result of fixed hereditary temporary connections of the type of instinctive complex chain reactions, together

---

[*] P.Ya.Gal'perin. Umstvennoe deistvie kak osnova formirovaniya mysli i obraza (Intellectual Activity as a Basis for the Formation of Thought and Image). — Voprosy Psikhologii, No. 6. 1957.

with the "natural" reflex coordinations which they involve, represent real automatism.*

In more highly developed vertebrates (mammals) the brain substrate of the voluntary as well as automatized direction is represented by the phylogenetically most recently developed neocortex with its highly complex and differentiated potentialities, and its anatomically multistratified structure (Figure 24), together with their connections with subcortical formations in the cerebral hemispheres and diencephalon (adjacent subcortex), and also with formations of the analyzing-coordinating system and the coordinating system localized below them (distant subcortex) (Figures 25 and 26).

We postulate that the fully developed new cortex contains the mechanism of direction which is related to the most highly developed stage in mammalian evolution, namely the frontal lobe of the brain.

In lower mammals this relatively little developed part of the brain represents mainly the motor zone of the cortex (Figure 24 A and B). In the more highly developed mammals, such as the carnivora (Figure 24C) and primates (Figure 24 D and E), this brain area is differentiated as the main cortical mechanism for effecting "voluntary", finely differentiated distinct movements (the motor cortex proper) and completely synthetized, elaborate movements (pre-motor cortical area). Both achieve a high degree of specialization in the higher mammals, i.e., in primates and particularly in man. In anthropoid apes possessing well developed cerebral hemispheres, comparable in shape to the human ones, the size of the frontal lobe increases considerably in connection with phylogenetic development of the more recent zones located in certain parts of the frontal lobe, and forming the actual frontal brain (Figure 24 E and F).

It has been established by A. R. Luriya** and his associates that the frontal lobe of the brain as a whole has a special significance for the organization of the total sphere of active voluntary activity in man; this is true from the simplest voluntary movements carried out through the motor cortex proper to the most complex manifestations of voluntary target-directed activity carried out with participation of the second signalling system, related to the frontal brain area proper. This part of the brain is concerned with carrying out particular patterns of behavior and comparison of results of purposeful activity. The significant role of a certain part of the motor zone of the cortex (pre-motor cortex — Figure 24, pm) in processes of automatization of voluntary movement has also been demonstrated.

The morphological basis of the higher organizers of behavior is represented by zones of the frontal area proper with their most complex mutual connections with cortical and subcortical representations of all analyzer systems, with representations of vital reactions in the brain, and with the mechanism of reflex coordinations located at lower levels of

---

* In contrast to our terminology which is based on the classification of different components of the function of direction, following evolutional biological patterns, Bernshtein also includes in the term automatisms those motor acts which are produced as a result of automatization of learned acquired reactions.

** A.R. Luriya. Vysshie korkovye funktsii cheloveka (Highest Cortical Functions in Man).— Izdatel'stvo MGU. 1962.
A.R. Luriya. Mozg cheloveka i psikhicheskie protsessy. Neiro-psikhologicheskie issledovaniya (The Human Brain and Mental Processes. Neuropsychologic Investigations).— Moskva, Izdatel'stvo APN RSFSR. 1963.

the CNS. In man, for example, these zones constitute a quarter of the total area of the new cortex.

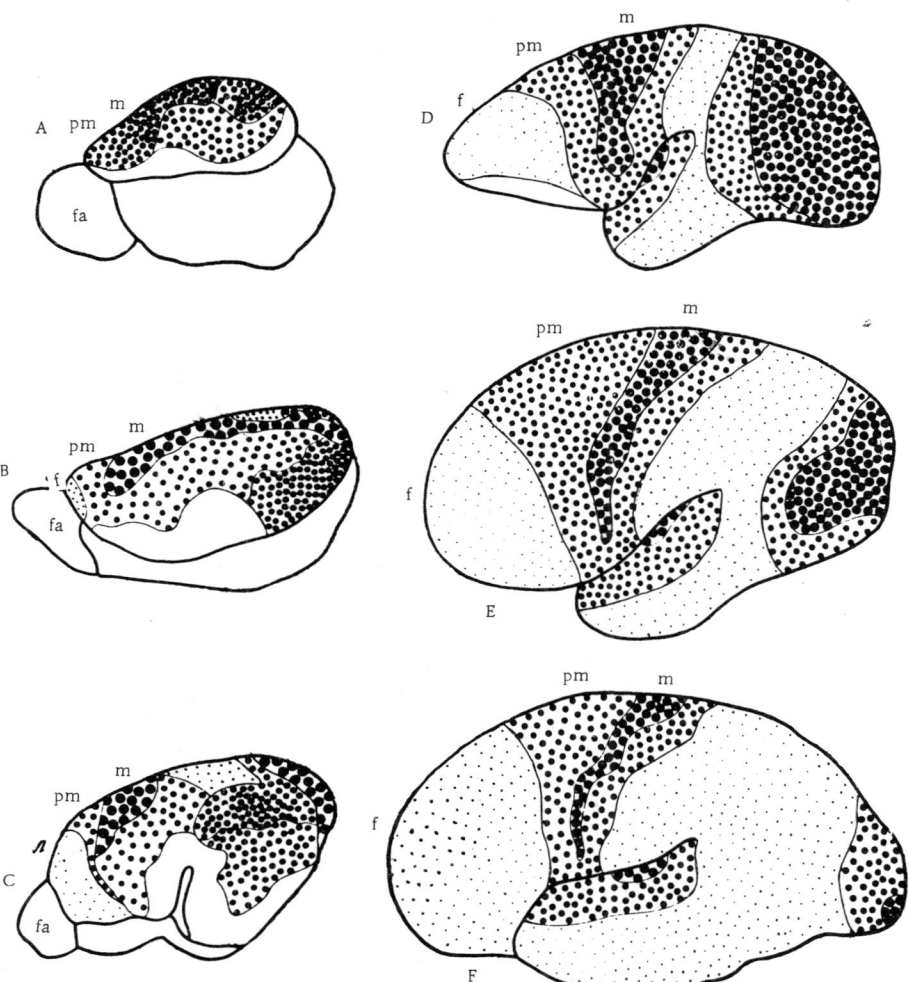

FIGURE 24. Schematic charts of progressive differentiation of cytoarchitectonic areas of various functional significance and of zones in the new cortex in a series of mammals:

A — hedgehog; B — rat; C — dog; D — lower apes; E — anthropoid apes; F — man; m — motor cortex proper (marked by large dotting); pm — pre-motor cortex (marked by medium-sized stippling); f — frontal area proper (marked by small stippling). Motor and pre-motor fields are included in the motor zone of the cortex. The motor zone and the frontal area [fa] together represent the frontal lobe of the brain (G. I. Polyakov, 1960).

During the past hundred years much literature has been devoted to describing the function and structure of the frontal lobe of the brain. We consider that "direction" defines most adequately the functional significance of this "powerful" part of the brain. The frontal lobe is that particular section of the entire CNS which in the course of animal evolution has specialized in carrying out the most complex forms of direction ("free," as well as automatized) with all their broad range of functions.

The clinical features of different types of injuries to the frontal lobe are manifested primarily by disorders of the various types of voluntary action. In the pathogenesis of these disorders there is some participation of defects in afferent syntheses taking place before initiation of the action, with the leading participation of frontal brain formations (A. R. Luriya). These disorders may also involve the disintegration of associated connections through which the functional interrelation of the highest forms of gnosis, praxis and speech are realized, and are conditioned by pathological changes in the most complex mental processes of perception, memory, thought and action.

A dissociation between intellectual, emotional and voluntary functions, as seen in schizophrenia, may be considered one of the most striking manifestations of functional disturbance of voluntary direction in brain lesions of the frontal cortex and its connections. In this particular disease, we believe the intellectual apparatus itself remains intact, but the patient loses the ability to use it adequately.

As already stated, impulses of voluntary and automatized direction are realized by means of numerous connections uniting the higher cortical centers of direction with all formations of the proximal and more distal subcortex, i.e., with the coordinating mechanism, the analyzing-coordinating mechanism and the nervous system centers responsible for autodirection. With the aid of such connections the cortical mechanism of direction is in a position to influence the effector instruments of the body in a more or less selective, differentiated way, depending on the degree of development of the effector sphere of the organism. A special pathway for the course of impulses of voluntary movements becomes differentiated during mammalian evolution, and achieves a particularly high degree of development in primates; this is the pyramidal tract connecting the motor and other areas of the cortex with the effector (motor) nuclei of the brain and spinal cord (Figure 25). This system of fibers has access to the effector neurons which provide direct innervation of the skeletal muscles of the entire body, as well as to the transmitting neurons of the reticular formations of the brain and spinal cord, i.e., to the elements of coordinating mechanism (see Figure 10B). It has also been established experimentally and morphologically that with higher degrees of organization in a series of mammals, the mechanism of direct influences of the cerebral cortex on the effector neurons becomes more and more prominent; this is manifested anatomically by an increase in the number of endings of the fibers of the pyramidal tract in the relevant neurons, together with endings directed to the transmitting neurons of the reticular formation.

The cerebral cortex exercises a constant excitatory or inhibitory effect on the state and activity of all subcortical reflex centers. In this activity, the motor cortex, which has direct connections with these centers, is of special significance. It has been determined that the cortical motor (pyramidal) tract is a source of constant bioelectric activity, through which the latent awareness of the reflex centers to stimuli is maintained and which aids in their rapid reaction. Additional influences originating in the cerebral cortex and acting on the autonomic nervous system centers ensure certain states of reacting organs (metabolism, blood supply, trophic processes), which aid in a more effective action of reflex potentials of the organism.

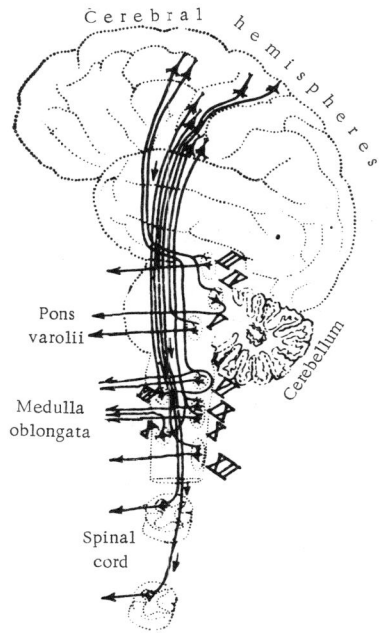 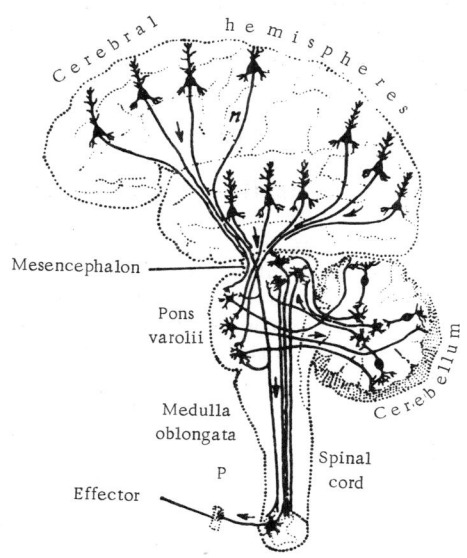

FIGURE 25. Pyramidal tract for transmission of impulses of direction from the cerebral cortex to the reflex centers of the brainstem and spinal cord included in the coordinating mechanism. Roman numerals mark the motor nuclei of the corresponding craniocerebral nerves. To simplify the diagram, the transmitting neurons of the reticular formation are not represented. (Modification according to V. M. Bekhterev.)

FIGURE 26. Diagram of extrapyramidal tracts acting as transmittors of impulses of direction from various areas of the cerebral cortex to the analyzing-coordinating mechanism (cerebellum). Diagram depicts the chain of consecutive transmissions of impulses from the cerebral cortex to the cerebellar cortex, and from there to the effector neurons:

p — pyramidal tract. (After Cajal, with some changes.)

Together with the pyramidal tracts providing direct connections to the higher cortical endings of the analyzer system with the corresponding sections of the coordinating mechanism, there is considerable development, especially in the CNS of higher animals, of the extrapyramidal tracts. These proceed from the cerebral cortex to the axial part of the CNS, and are directed mainly to various formations of the analyzing-coordinating mechanism. In primates, in view of their arboreal mode of life and upright walk, the most important of these tracts are connections with the cerebellum, originating in the various areas of the new cortex (Figure 26). The fibers of the pyramidal tract bypassing the analyzing-coordinating mechanism also yield numerous collaterals to corresponding groups of neurons distributed on different levels of the CNS.

The extrapyramidal connections of the cortex with the analyzing-coordinating formations (especially with the cerebellum) play quite a significant role in the processes of automatization of voluntary motor acts. It could be assumed that in animals the mechanisms of regulation and control are no less important in automatization of voluntary movements and actions. Anatomically, this means that realization of formulae of transmission of effector activities, from voluntary to involuntary-automatized, performed in the cortical endings of the analyzer systems (transciphering, according to Bernshtein), depends to a considerable degree on those collateral connections, through which the analyzer systems act on the mechanisms of reflex coordinations, along the axial part of the CNS.

Impulses of voluntary direction "initiating" the chain reaction of automatization reach the different components of autoregulating and autocontrolling formation with a degree of "penetrability" which is not uniform. Automatic reflex coordinations, which include primarily autoregulation of internal activities of the body, are little or not at all subject to external influences, in contrast to consciously directed reflex processes. Experiments conducted in the laboratory of E. A. Asratyan have established that participation of the cerebral cortex in compensatory processes connected with impaired activity of the internal organs is expressed to a lesser degree than when related to reflex activities directed to the outside.

We assume that the forms of direction discussed above may be reproduced by means of an experimental technical model. The constructor of such a model must therefore reproduce a block of automatic direction with fixed programs of behavior included in it, then a block of direction proper, supposing the ability of the machine to teach with subsequent automatization of learned (acquired) activities.

8. PSYCHOPHYSIOLOGICAL ASPECTS OF THE MECHANISM OF DIRECTION

The prospect of studying the actual interrelations of different forms of direction in the animal organism is quite promising both from the physiological and the psychophysiological point of view. The field of problems examined here may, in fact, include all those psychological problems associated with the organization of a planned purposeful activity, the anticipation of the likelihood of occurrence of definite events (with special reference to extrapolated reflexes investigated by L. V. Krushinskii*), interrelations of voluntary and involuntary, conscious and unconscious aspects of active mental acts, and internal interactions of voluntary, intellectual and emotional functions.

---

* L. V. Krushinskii. Izuchenie ekstrapolyatsionnykh refleksov u zhivotnykh (Study of Extrapolated Reflexes in Animals).— In: Problemy kibernetiki, No. 2, Moskva, Fizmatgiz. 1959.
L. V. Krushinskii. Formirovanie povedeniya zhivotnykh v norme i patologii (Formation of Normal and Pathological Behavior in Animals).— Izdatel'stvo MGU. 1960.

The interrelations of the conscious (voluntary) and unconscious (involuntary) functions are apparently of considerable value for understanding all aspects of the complex problem of direction. We proceed in this from the observations and experiments of G. V. Gershuni* and others, who have studied subsensory reactions to subthreshold stimuli, and have shown the presence of hidden subconscious courses of processes of brain activity, preceding the appearance of mental acts reflected in consciousness: feelings, perceptions, logical intellectual conclusions and purposeful actions. Such unacknowledged processes, i. e., processes which according to our concept have already passed the stage of primary automatization ("mental automatisms," according to P. Zhane), act as a particular outline formed during individual ontogeny, which holds the entire chain of cause-and-effect connections between successive stages of various voluntary actions.

Bernshtein's theory on coordinating levels, as already mentioned, is closely related to the problem of interrelations of the conscious and unconscious in the function of direction. In any complex voluntary act, only that part which is related to the guiding level of the action carried out reaches consciousness. All other supporting ("background") factors participate as unconscious components of the performed action, i. e., remain in the shade, so to speak, outside the limits of the "bright field" of consciousness. The function which must be carried out is fixed in consciousness but not the means of accomplishing the corresponding actions (practical and intellectual). Only the logical sequence of the accomplished actions come to conscious awareness, and not their separate components.

It must be added that no voluntary human action becomes uniformly clearly conscious at all stages of its initiation or course. The stimulus provoking the action, and completion of the action, as a concrete expression of achievement (or nonachievement) of the task to which the given action is directed, enter consciousness most clearly, as a rule.

The various stages of a voluntary act and the conscious awareness of them are apparently very complex, both on the methodological and methodical plane; how this occurs is still far from clear. Various voluntarily accomplished acts apparently differ greatly in the number of their components which can be represented simultaneously in consciousness.

This definition of "automatized direction" does not exhaust by any means all the possibilities of realization of direction in an unconscious way. For example, hypnotic suggestion may apparently be considered as such a particular psychophysiological condition, when the activity of the higher centers of direction is transferred from the conscious to the subconscious level, while the formal structure underlying the performance of the operation is fully preserved. It is known that hypnotized persons are able to retain even the most complicated instructions in their memory for varying periods, and although these remain in the subconscious, they can nevertheless be carried out with precision. It follows that there may be modes of direction in which the entire reaction directed from the cerebral cortex proceeds from beginning to end without a clear realization of the signaling significance of the initiating stimulus and the sense of its effect.

---

* G. V. Gershuni. Reflektornye reaktsii pri vozdeistvii vneshnikh razdrazhenii na organy chuvstv cheloveka i ikh svyazi s oshchushcheniyami (Reflex Reactions during Action of External Stimuli on Sense Organs of Man in their Connection with Sensations). — Fiziologicheskii Zhurnal SSSR, Vol. 35, No. 5. 1949.

Another example of the great functional complexity of human direction is provided by the dual psychophysiological state of an actor, connected with a particular distribution of consciousness and attention during the process of stage activity. An actor playing on the stage (according to K. S. Stanislavskii's system) must be capable, through continuous preliminary training, to evoke various experiences, moods or emotions at will, while remaining unaffected by them, in contrast to natural behavior in life. One great actor has defined this as a state of preparedness of the body to obey any order dictated by thought or will; an actor is his own master as well as master of the various roles he portrays.

The following series of experiments to which P. S. Kupalov refers may serve as a good illustration of the problem of the mechanism of the voluntary induction of involuntary reactions in animals.

A conditioned reflex was formed in a dog to the tapping of a metronome. The dog had to jump onto a table where the feed box was. Coming down from the table the dog usually shook himself. If at that moment the metronome sounds, followed by food intake, a functional connection is established between the involuntary reaction of shaking and the sound of the metronome indicating the presence of food. This resulted in the dog's shaking more and more often — up to 12 times per experiment. After a year the animal could perform this actively involuntary movement so easily and precisely that it gave the impression of a "voluntary" motor act.

One may assume that there are three stories of interrelations of conscious and unconscious components in the integral function of direction. Each of these stories is characterized by its particular level, or degree of submission of the unconscious components to the conscious ones.

The lowest level in this respect, formed during the earliest stage of development of the animal organism, is represented in animals of greater complexity by influences of involuntary character undoubtedly exerted by the higher sections of the encephalon on the total autonomic sphere of the organism. We are referring to influences of the cerebral cortex on the most intimate processes of the internal life of the body. States of affect, suggestion or hypnosis are, for instance, accompanied by changes in the blood sugar level (K. I. Platonov*).

The next experiment can serve as an illustration of these types of influence. In a dog with an unimpaired CNS the composition of the gastric juice is altered according to the type of food ingested. Following removal of the cerebral cortex there is no difference in juice secretion; the animal secretes the same juice with intake of different foods.

It is perfectly clear that the most deeply hidden form of direction mentioned above takes its course, from beginning to end, as a process that is completely unconscious and quite independent of will. The role of the voluntary component in this case is almost nonexistent. In other words, the liberation of the involuntary component from the authority of the voluntary one is expressed to a maximal degree.

The physical substrate of such "hidden" cortical influences, achieving great power in some mental states, is probably related to the mechanism

---

* K.I. Platonov. Slovo kak fiziologicheskii i lechebnyi faktor (The Word as a Physiological and Therapeutic Factor). — Moskva, Medgiz. 1962. Third edition.

of connections of the corresponding formations of the new cortex with the phylogenetically older cortical and subcortical formations of the hypothalamus and the reticular formations in the brainstem.

The middle level, which can also be characterized as a transition from the lower level to the highest, is represented by a form of direction in which the involuntary-unconscious is only partly subjected to the voluntary-conscious. Such an interrelation of the components in the different variations is present in the emotional sphere, to be exact, in the influences exerted by the cerebral cortex on the senses, moods and degree of "intensity" of experiences. Diverse emotional manifestations are usually produced involuntarily in the depths of the subconscious, but are to a certain degree accessible to voluntary influences, i. e., they may be surpressed, restrained, or, on the contrary, intensified.

Finally, the highest level, formed latest in animal evolution and gaining full prominence only in the stage of development of man, is related mainly to movements and actions carried out at will. At this stage of differentiation of the physical mechanism of consciousness, the involuntary components are subjected to a maximum degree to the voluntary ones. This category of involuntary and unconscious components of voluntary acts can include fully the concept of automatized direction in its broadest aspect, as we formulated earlier, i. e., keeping in mind automatization not only of actions but also of logical processes.

As already mentioned, the motor acts performed are excluded from the sphere of continuously existing consciousness and are transferred to the level of automatized processes.

The highest level of the function of direction almost certainly also includes the various intellectual activities in the formation and realization of which the participation of both voluntary and involuntary (automatized) components may be assumed to take place. Not only motor acts, but also intellectual function (perception, thoughts, and memory) can be automatized to some degree, and be carried out below the threshold of consciousness. The "unconscious (mental) deductions" described by Helmholtz may be part of these phenomena

In some situations presenting increased demands for rapidity of the processes of perception and intelligence, such psychophysiological mechanisms acquire special significance. The profession of a pilot directing a jet requires a most rapid, quick-as-lightning orientation, reasoning and decision. According to the cosmonaut G. S. Titov's statement, "specialized automatisms" must be perfected by the present-day fighter pilot, who must combine thought to "mix" with action; in the very instance in which this takes place it is "difficult to establish what comes first, action or judgment."

One may assume that one of the major trends in further progress of human nature and the central nervous organization includes a more functional improvement of the cerebral apparatus of direction. This process may serve as a natural prerequisite of man's further mastering not only of external phenomena but also of the self, through the potential reflex possibilities inherent in his physical make-up, and directed to ever-increasing submission to voluntary direction of those parts of reflex activity which are presently still independent, or subject to such direction to a minor degree only. In this connection it is appropriate to refer to an expression of Pavlov. With his particular ability to pinpoint the substance of various problems, Pavlov wrote that understanding the nature of instincts "will help us to understand ourselves and to develop the capacity for personal autodirection within ourselves."

9. INTERRELATIONS OF THE FUNCTIONS OF AUTO-REGULATION, AUTOCONTROL AND AUTODIRECTION FROM THE EVOLUTIONARY POINT OF VIEW

In the lower multicellular animal organisms with a primitive neuronal construction (Coelenterata, Echinodermata), the ability to direct behavior, in the real sense of the word, is apparently scarcely developed. Such organisms represent a type of living automatons, highly perfected in the "technical" sense, but capable of realizing only primitive forms of adaptations to changes in the environment. The elementary character of their reactions is based on the fact that these reactions are direct responses to stimuli acting at the given moment. These beings are unable to "calculate" situation changes likely to occur as results of their reactions. In other words, they do not yet possess centralized behavior. Their existence takes its course as if in momentary sections of space-time.

The noncentralized reticular system of the Coelenterata does not show signs of cephalization, i.e., there is no "cephalic" component in it; it can be defined as having little autocontrol and even less autodirection. Basically, this primitive type of neuron structure, capable of carrying out coordinated reactions to adequate stimuli, works on the principle of an autoregulated mechanism. I. Uexküll* compares graphically the totality of reactions of an echinoderm (sea urchin and starfish) to a "republic of reflexes." One may assume that the reflex possibilities of the animal under discussion surpass the elementary coordinating mechanism to a slight degree only.

The lower Metazoa, which have as yet a poorly developed "spontaneous" activity and insufficient ability to react in a directed manner to nature, nevertheless disclose a certain variety of precisely delineated, even if primitive, reflex coordinations connected with ecological factors acting on them.

A necessary anatomical-physiological prerequisite for the development of autocontrol and autodirection functions is the differentiation of a special central section within the neuronal structure, which interprets the information received by the various sense organs, and synthesizes more complex patterns of reaction. This type of a central nervous system component is the encephalon, which begins to be differentiated during the stage of the nerve cord system in lower worms. It may be said of this stage, when there is already a primitive degree of centralization of neurons, that it leads to the development of early types of analyzers. The cerebral "board" of control and direction (in the broad sense) begins to be more clearly discernible in invertebrates which have accomplished the transition from aquatic to terrestrial environment, and which possess an already more complex organized ganglionic nervous system (annelids).

In higher invertebrates such as crustaceans, insects and Cephalopoda there are already initial analyzers represented by certain formations in

---

* I. Uexküll. Theoretische Biologie, Berlin. 1928. Second edition.

their cerebrum. Concerning these animals, we can speak of functions of autocontrol and autoregulation with some elementary components of direction, which are sufficiently clearly defined, even if primitive in comparison with those in vertebrates. Such functions are related to different sections of their cerebral ganglia. The subpharyngeal ganglia (see Figure 2) which we consider as representing the elementary analyzing-coordinating system, are concerned mainly with autocontrol; the suprapharyngeal ganglia, which are concerned with registering the reprocessing stimuli (referable to smell, sight, etc.) and the integration of external perceptions with internal factors affecting the organism, carry out the function of autoregulation.

In the comparative series of invertebrates once can observe an increase in the ability of the brain to act in a guiding manner (stimulating or inhibiting) on different reflex coordinations of the nerve cord. However, real "organizing" prerequisites for the rapid progress of development of the function of "free" direction appear in vertebrates only. We discover directions developed to a greater or lesser degree only in these representatives of the animal world possessing, in comparison with invertebrates, a highly complex organized nervous system in the form of a nerve cord with a most advanced cephalization. The lateral ramifications of this branch of the evolutionary tree (fish and birds) have developed an adaptation to the environment mainly by means of autoregulation.

To summarize, one may say that differentiation of the general plan of neuronal structure in phylogenesis is based on the principle of triple co-subordination with reliance on interactions of the functions of autoregulation, autocontrol and autodirection.

In animal evolution several steps may be defined which reflect the different stages of organization of behavior.

The lowest level of development includes all above-mentioned functions still united in a single common complex, in which the function of autoregulation, which forms earliest in evolution, has the role of a "leader."

In the lowest Metazoa (Coelenterata, Echinodermata) this function is dominant in the orientation, nutrition, defense and adaptation reactions, and in the completion of temporary connections. The principle of autoregulation, with its underlying anatomical-physiological coordinating mechanism, appears at these stages as a determining factor on which the development of reflex adaptations depends.

In the subsequent evolutional stages the function of autoregulation is concentrated in the lower axial sections of the centralized nervous system, both in higher invertebrates and in all vertebrates. The reflex adaptations realized through the coordinating mechanism may be considered as autoregulating components of a completing process, as well as of orienting, adaptive and other vitally important reactions. It must be mentioned in particular that manifestations of total effect, and of dominants related to the coordinating mechanism, appear in the capacity of this type of component of the completing function. According to our concept, all elements of formation of reflex coordination and completion of temporary connections still act together.

In the most primitive vertebrates (Cyclostomata) the coordinating mechanism apparently still plays a basic role in reflex adaptations, since the analyzing-coordinating formations and supraaxial CNS are relatively poorly represented in these animals. Accordingly, the functions of autocontrol and autodirection take place on a primitive level.

With the development of analyzers constituting the physical substrate for higher functional possibilities of the animal organism, autocontrol, compared with autoregulation, gains in functional significance. It apparently is at its peak in the lower vertebrates (fishes) which have complex differentiated analyzing-coordinating formations of the axial part of the CNS, while the highest supraaxial part is still relatively poorly developed (see Figure 6). It follows that we may speak at this stage of autocontrolled components of completion of temporary connection (i.e., those which take place with the participation of lower cerebral parts of analyzers) and also of orientation, adaptation and other reflexes. These animals seem to have adapted definitively to their environment.

The components of the completing function acting at axial levels of the CNS were described in a series of experiments (A. I. Karamyan*) indicating the significant role of the cerebellum in the development of conditioned reflexes in lower vertebrates.

The progressively more marked domination of direction later in evolution (with its auxiliaries in the form of regulation and control) coincides with further development and differentiation of the analyzers. The most significant changes in the CNS of mammals are closely connected with the structural and functional differentiation of the analyzer systems, particularly their highest (supraaxial) cerebral components. The cerebral mechanisms of direction proper are first fully developed in primates.

This stage of phylogenesis is marked by an increasingly greater role in direction, control and regulation in reflex coordinations of the axial part of the CNS; in the lateral ramifications of this branch of the evolutionary tree, represented by fish and birds, autodirection is of primary importance. Formation of the most highly organized components of environmental orientation and adaptation occur with the participation of these functions; it is manifested by active motor adjustments to stimuli received by the analyzer systems. This forms the basis for the physiological mechanism of attention and apperception. Actually, the activity of the cortical part of the completing apparatus becomes more intricately and finely differentiated. This process provides wide possibilities for expansion of the organism's individual reflex domination not only of its past and present but also of its future.

---

* A. I. Karamyan. Evolyutsiya funktsii mozzhechka i bol'shikh polusharii (Evolution of the Function of the Cerebellum and the Cerebral Hemispheres). — Leningrad, Medgiz. 1956.

Chapter III

THE NEURON NETWORK

1. ORIGIN AND DIFFERENTIATION OF THE NEURON NETWORK

Even complicated things may be basically very simple. However, the investigator attempting to understand the elementary principles on which even highly complex manifestations are based may be confronted with considerable difficulties. In order to overcome them, a theory or hypothesis must first exist to provide a valid explanation of certain facts observed, and these must be tested and verified experimentally.

In that branch of science studying brain function, as in other fields of the natural sciences, comparative-historical, evolutionary methods of analysis and synthesis of accumulated facts are of major importance. The comparative study of topographic interrelations and structure of neurons, and specific features of their connections in the peripheral subcortical and cortical components of the analyzers, is essential; this, and the study of connections of various components by conduction pathways at the various stages of vertebrate evolution, provide information on some morphological criteria which determine the complexity of the structure as a whole.

In our understanding of the origin, development, continuing differentiation and perfection of the structure of the brain, which provides a physical basis of interrelations within the organism and between the organism and the external world, we proceed from two basic premises.

The basic pattern of neuron structure derives from the biological principle of multiple interconnections of all stimuli-perceiving elements (receptors) with all the organism's elements effecting responses to these stimuli (effectors). Any receptor, or combination of receptors, can be connected with any effector, or combination of effectors. This principle is represented anatomically by a rich network of nerve pathways uniting the various specific receptor points of the body, or their groups, with effectors (Figure 27A). As will be shown in Chapter IV, a similar principle is applied in the geometric construction of transmitting links, and the conductors connecting these links in the analyzers, and especially in the complex analyzer systems.

The inherent capacity of the animal organism to adjust by reflex reaction of broad range and great variety to a constantly changing environment, and a potential ability to react to all possible combinations of external and internal stimuli, is expressed in the general functional connection of receptors with effectors, arranged in this manner in the brain matter.

Our second premise, stemming directly from the former, is concerned with the structural differentiation of all elements of reflex action. It makes use of the hypothesis that neurons represent an apparatus connecting receptors and effectors, and are formed not by chance, but by conforming to a certain law at the points of intersection of pathways passing from receptors to effectors in the body.

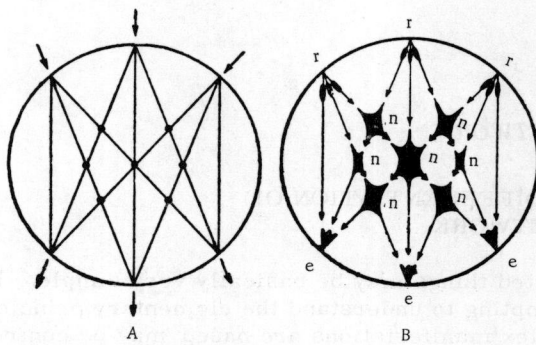

FIGURE 27

A — Diagram of the "network" of distribution of nerve impulse pathways from the receptor (upper arrows) to the effector (lower arrows) points of the body.

B — Diagram of an elementary network of neurons, illustrating the origin of neurons at junctional points connecting receptors with effectors. The direction of nerve impulse transmission is indicated by arrows:

r — receptor; e — effector; n — neuron.

As seen in Figure 27B the neurons originate and become structurally reinforced at the points of intersection of nerve impulses of different origin and designation. Thus the neuron, from the very beginning of its appearance in animal evolution, functions as an apparatus of convergence and separation of impulses transmitted through it. One may assume that in actively functioning nervous systems (possibly with rare exceptions) all neurons are coordinated to act according to such a principle. The convergence of different types of nerve impulses in certain neurons, and their subsequent divergence, has been clearly demonstrated in different formations of the CNS: in the cerebral cortex, subcortical formations (optic thalamus, subcortical ganglia of the cerebral hemispheres, and the complex of the amygdaloid nuclei) and reticular formations of the brainstem. The convergence of different afferent impulses on effector (motor) neurons, which Sherrington has compared to a "funnel", is one particular example. N. A. Bernshtein has compared the synthesis of many impulses entering from various CNS levels and acting on the motor neuron with the performance of a number of musicians playing with one bow on a single cello.

In the course of progressive centralization of the nervous system, accompanied by increasing predominance of the brain over the spinal cord (cephalization) and concomitant with the increasing complexity of interaction of neurons, marked changes take place in the neuron network; these involve the structure of neurons and the total system of interneuron connections.

They are manifest in reinforcement of the terminal branches of the peripheral afferent nerve fibers (see Figure 1) conducting impulses from receptors with the cytoplasmic processes (dendrites) typical of the nerve cells. At the same time there is an increase in the number of branchings (collaterals) emerging from nerve fibers, or axons, of nerve cells included in the centralized nervous system itself.

As a result of these improvements in neuronal structure, more and more close and differentiated contacts form between the various neurons participating together in carrying out certain reflex reactions; they also aid in completion of circuits of reverse connections in the process of transmission of impulses in reflex arcs. This underlies the anatomical-physiological mechanism of continuous retention in the nerve centers of the traces of incoming stimuli and the reproduction of resulting reaction patterns. In the analyzers, and especially in their cortical components, these characteristics of neuron structure attain the most elaborate degree of differentiation, as compared with other parts of the CNS (see Chapter IV, Section 2).

2. PROGRESSIVE DIFFERENTIATION OF NEURONS

In the less highly developed vertebrates, the CNS is still relatively little differentiated (Figure 28A). Neurons receiving impulses from the periphery, transmitting them to various parts of the CNS and converting them to impulses transmitted back, are still functionally indistinctly differentiated. From their structural features, these elements can be characterized as elements intermediate between effector and reticular neurons, and possessing some properties of both. In subsequent stages of evolution these primitive coordinating mechanisms acquire a higher degree of specialization and a spatial separation of neurons of different functional significance. This process occurs in the following three main directions (Figure 28B).

On the one hand, there is a separation between the executive part of the coordinating system, represented by groups of effector (motor) neurons (Figure 28B, 3) which innervate the motor and secretory organs of the body directly. On the other hand, separate groups of special transmitting neurons are assigned to adjust for coordination of interactions of effector neurons included in the local segmental reflex mechanisms distributed along the axial part of the CNS.

As already mentioned in Chapter I (see Section 3), the aggregates of these neurons (Figure 28B, 4), which constitute the suprasegmental part of the coordinating mechanism, produce the reticular formation of the spinal cord and brainstem. The reticular neurons are included in the local reflex arcs in the capacity of intermediate supplementary links of transmissions of centripetal afferent impulses entering the CNS from corresponding receptors, and are subsequently distributed among the various motor nerve centers. These elements, together with the returning collaterals emerging from the axons of the effector nerve cells, play a particularly important role in the completion of circuits of returning connections (see Figure 43 B and D) in the reflex arcs of the spinal cord and brainstem, and are of significance in the coordinating systems of different reflexes.

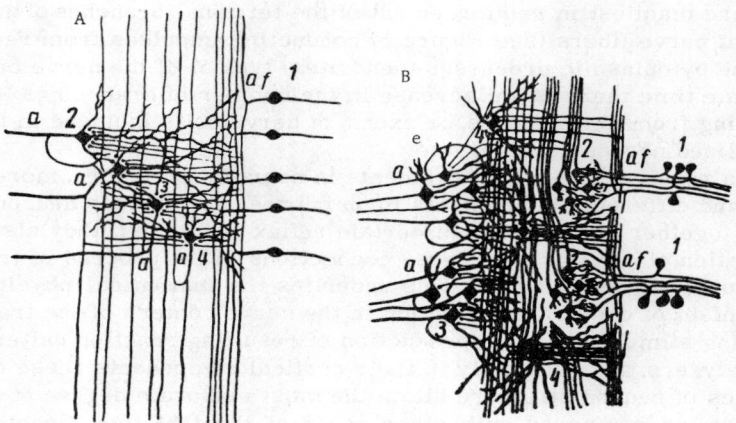

FIGURE 28. Neuron structure of the CNS:

A — of a lower vertebrate: 1 — peripheral sensory neurons; 2, 3, 4 — central neurons of a mixed type which later differentiate into effector (motor) and reticular neurons (see B); af — peripheral afferent fibers; a — axon neurons (G. I. Poliakov, 1959);
B — of a higher vertebrate: ganglia of neuron transmission along the pathways of analyzers; e — effector (motor) neurons; 1, 2, 3 — as in diagram A; 4 — reticular neurons; af and a — as in diagram A (G. I. Poliakov, 1959).

The development of analyzers represents, as we know, a further step in the process of CNS organization, together with more detailed differentiation of groups of effectors and reticular neurons which are a part of local coordinating reflex apparatuses. Analyzer systems are formed as an apparatus for the execution and transmission of a closely concentrated flow of centripetal nervous impulses.

The main body of elements of which the transmitting ganglia are formed, linked together in a single continuous analyzer system, consists of afferent neurons (Figure 29) conducting impulses to the succeeding transmitting link of the chain. The axons of these nerve cells terminate in the transmitting station which they enter as afferent fibers.

The efferent neurons of analyzers (Figure 30C) differ typically at all levels of transmission, from the effector (Figure 30A) and reticular neurons (Figure 30B), in the denser ramification of the dendrite clusters emerging from the bodies of the nerve cells. The endings of the effector fibers, linked with dendrites of efferent neurons and presenting a typical "bubble" or "grape cluster" form, also possess a large number of ramifications. Another feature worth noting of the transmitting apparatus in analyzers is the considerable development of lateral and returning collaterals in axons of efferent neurons, which form the main pathways for transmission of centripetal stimuli.

These particular features of the structure of transmitting ganglia in analyzers are evidently conditioned by the dense concentration of transmitted impulses and complexity of changes they undergo during the process of transfer from certain groups of neurons to others.

This concept of the structure of elements of analyzers and their interrelations has also been described in physiological experiments

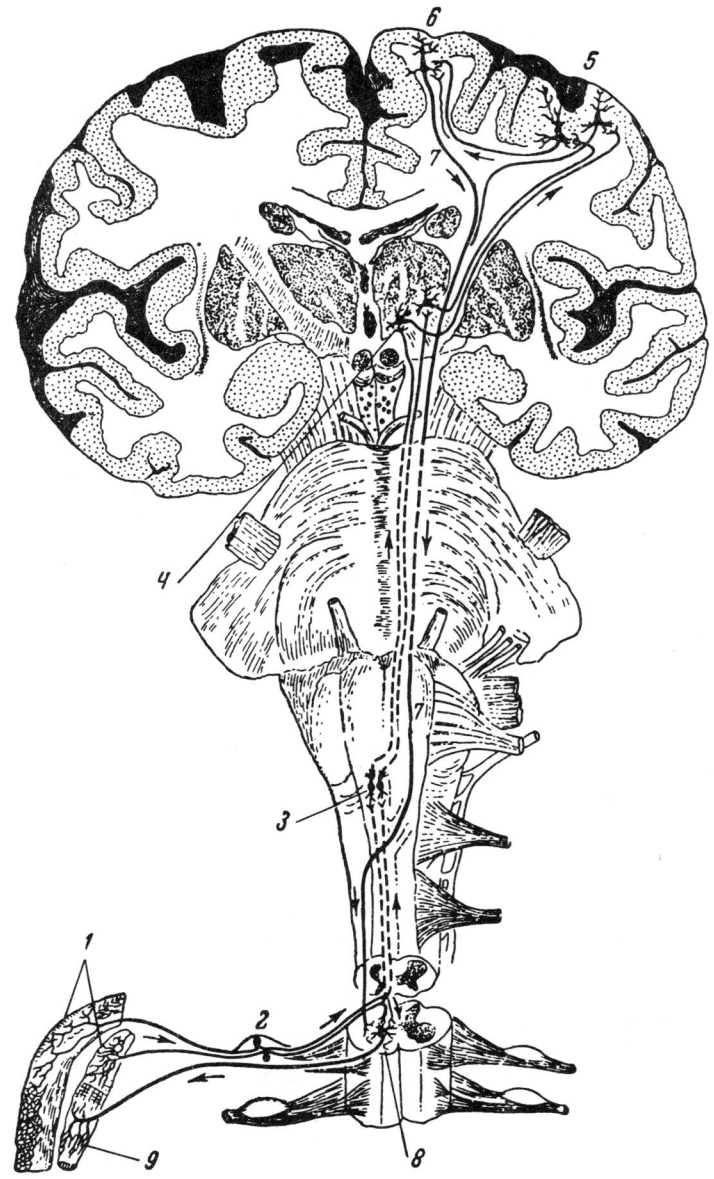

FIGURE 29. Systems of skin and kinesthetic analyzers (transmitting impulses from motor organs). Represented are long-axon efferent neurons:

1 — endings of sensory nerve fibers in the skin and motor organs (muscles);
2 — peripheral sensory neurons of intervertebral ganglia; 3 — transmitting nuclei in the medulla oblongata; 4 — transmitting (relay) nuclei in the optic thalamus; 5 — dermatokinesthetic (general sensory) zone of the cortex; 6 — motor zone of the cortex; 7 — pathway from the motor cortex to the motor centers of the brain and spinal cord (pyramidal tract); 8 — effector (motor) neuron of the spinal cord; 9 — motor neuron terminals in the skeletal muscles (G.I. Poliakov, 1956).

(R. A. Durinyan*). The electrophysiological method (of registering so-called induced potentials) has been used to demonstrate some significant functional topographic correlations of groups conducting and transmitting impulses of elements present in analyzers. In the conducting pathways and transmitting centers along the analyzer systems sections can be distinguished in which nerve fibers and neuron cells are particularly close together. At the points at which clusters of nerve fibers and nerve cells are most dense, bioelectric potentials (so-called foci of maximal bioelectric activity) are most typically registered following stimulation of corresponding sections of sensitive areas or nerves.

The dense concentration of nervous elements in foci of maximal activity create conditions favorable for a synchronized discharge of many elements. Electrophysiologically, this process is manifest in a minimal latent period with a maximal amplitude of the induced potential. In those sections of the CNS (e.g., in the reticular formation of the brainstem and "non-specific" nuclei of the optic thalamus in its continuation) and where neuron transmissions are less densely distributed, the foci of maximal activity are not so much in evidence.

3. SPECIAL TRANSMITTING NEURONS AND THEIR SIGNIFICANCE IN REFLEX ACTIVITY

Special intermediate or intercalated neurons are found to act as additional or auxiliary elements in the chain of direct transfer of impulses along the pathways of segmental reflex arcs and analyzers. Such elements are represented in local reflex systems of the spinal cord and brainstem by reticular neurons mentioned earlier (see Figure 3, rn; Figure 7, rn; Figure 9, stn; Figure 14, rn). The main difference between the reticular neurons and the effectors consists in the absence of a direct termination of reticular neurons at the periphery; they distribute their processes inside the corresponding CNS sections, while the effector neurons, always present at terminal points of the CNS, project their axons to the periphery, i.e., to the corresponding muscles and glands.

Investigations during recent years have tended to confirm the fact that even the most elementary reflexes affected by simple two-neuron reflex arcs proceed regularly only with participation of special transmitting neurons; the latter are represented in the CNS by reticular nerve elements (see Figure 10 B, 3). Even more important are the elements which we relate to the general group of special transmitting neurons in the processes of coordinating interaction and transfer of impulses to the analyzing-coordinating mechanism and in the analyzer systems. The presence of these elements at points of transmission of impulses in analyzer pathways was confirmed in morphological and electrophysiological studies (J. Eccles,** P.G. Kostyuk †). Neurons which in response to a single stimulus generate

---

* R.A. Durinyan. Osnovnye cherty tsentral'noi organizatsii vistseral'nykh afferentnykh sistem (Eksperimental'nyi elektrograficheskii analiz) (Main Features of the Central Organization of Visceral Afferent Systems (Experimental Electrographic Analysis)). – Doctoral Thesis. Moskva. 1963.

** J. Eccles. Physiology of Nerve Cells. – John Hopkins Press. 1957.

† P.G. Kostyuk. Izuchenie funktsional'nykh osobennostei razlichnykh tsentral'nykh neironov pri pomoshchi vnutrikletochnykh mikroelektrodov (A Study of the Functional Features of Central Neurons with the Aid of Intracellular Microelectrodes). – Moskva, Medgiz. 1962.

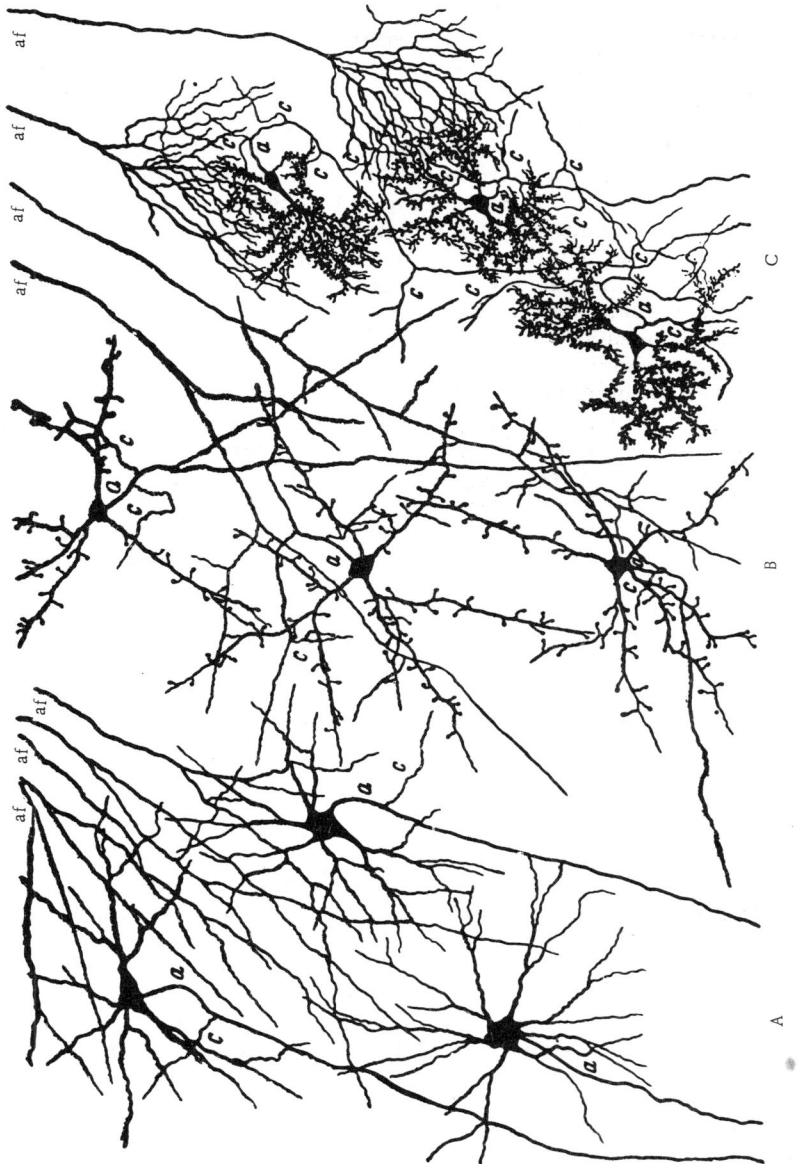

FIGURE 30. Characteristic structural features of neurons and afferent fibers in motor (effector) nuclei (A), nuclei of the reticular formation (B) and transmitting nuclei of analyzers (C):

af — afferent fibers; a — axons of nerve cells; c — initial (lateral and returning) collaterals of axons. Note clusters of dendritic branches in the transmitting stations of analyzers.

discharges of frequencies of 1,000 cs and more were found in the relay nuclei of kinesthetic and skin analyzers present in the medulla oblongata and later also in the cerebral cortex and other brain areas. As mentioned (see Chapter I, Section 3), rhythmic high-frequency discharges to a single stimulus are typical of reactions of special transmitting neurons.

We distinguished two types of elements in the special transmitting neurons. It was first noted that typical neurons possessing few dendrites (see Figure 30B) from the surrounding reticular formation penetrate groups of efferent neurons with a dense dendritic branching (Figure 30C), together forming ganglia of transmission elements in the analyzers (G.P. Zhukova and T.A. Leontovich, 1964). Similar structures in the same locations were described by other authors (M. E. Scheibel and A. B. Scheibel*), who were unable to identify them as neurons of the reticular formation.

Reticular-type neurons are found in nuclei of the posterior horns of the spinal cord (Figure 31A), in sensory nuclei of craniocerebral nerves and transmitting nuclei of analyzers located in the medulla oblongata (Figure 31B); they are also present in formations of the lower parts of the subcortex, serving as transit stations along the pathways of transfer of centripetal impulses to the cerebral cortex, in the relay nuclei of the optic thalamus (Figure 31C) and in the medial and lateral geniculate bodies.

The presence of reticular-type neurons in the analyzing-coordinating mechanism and in analyzer systems is not surprising. It is evidently conditioned by the fact that these elements are of significant value in correlation and functional connections established between analyzers and the coordinating mechanism proper, in reactions of the organism to impulses entering from its external and internal environment.

An estimate of the structural complexity of the analyzers is provided by the fact that interspersed among the reticular neurons (Figure 32, A and B) other transmitting elements are to be found, such as short-axon neurons (transitional forms) (Figure 32, C and D). Elements of one or another type are distributed in the main body of efferent neurons transmitting centripetal impulses along the analyzer.

The main difference between reticular neurons and neurons with short axons is as follows. Reticular neurons have an axon of varying length, and this with its ramifications runs along the CNS axis, forming contacts with groups of effectors or other reticular neurons, located in different segments of the spinal cord or at various levels of the brainstem (Figure 32, A and B; Figure 14, rn). On the other hand, as K. Golgi and R. Cajal, who were the first to describe neuron structure, have already noted, the short-axon neurons do not, as a rule, exceed the limits of a relatively restricted section of the gray matter, where the cell itself is found; the terminal branches of the short-axon neurons are distributed in the bodies and dendrites of neighboring cells (see Figure 42 x — stellate cells with short axons in layer IV of the cerebral cortex).

Interneuron connections, established through special transmitting neurons with axons of varying length, play an important role in the regular activity of various groups of efferent neurons. During the process of transmission of impulses from afferent to efferent neurons, elements of

---

* M.E. Scheibel and A.B. Scheibel. The Inferior Olivary Peduncle. — "Journ. Comp. Neurol." 102, No. 1. 1955.

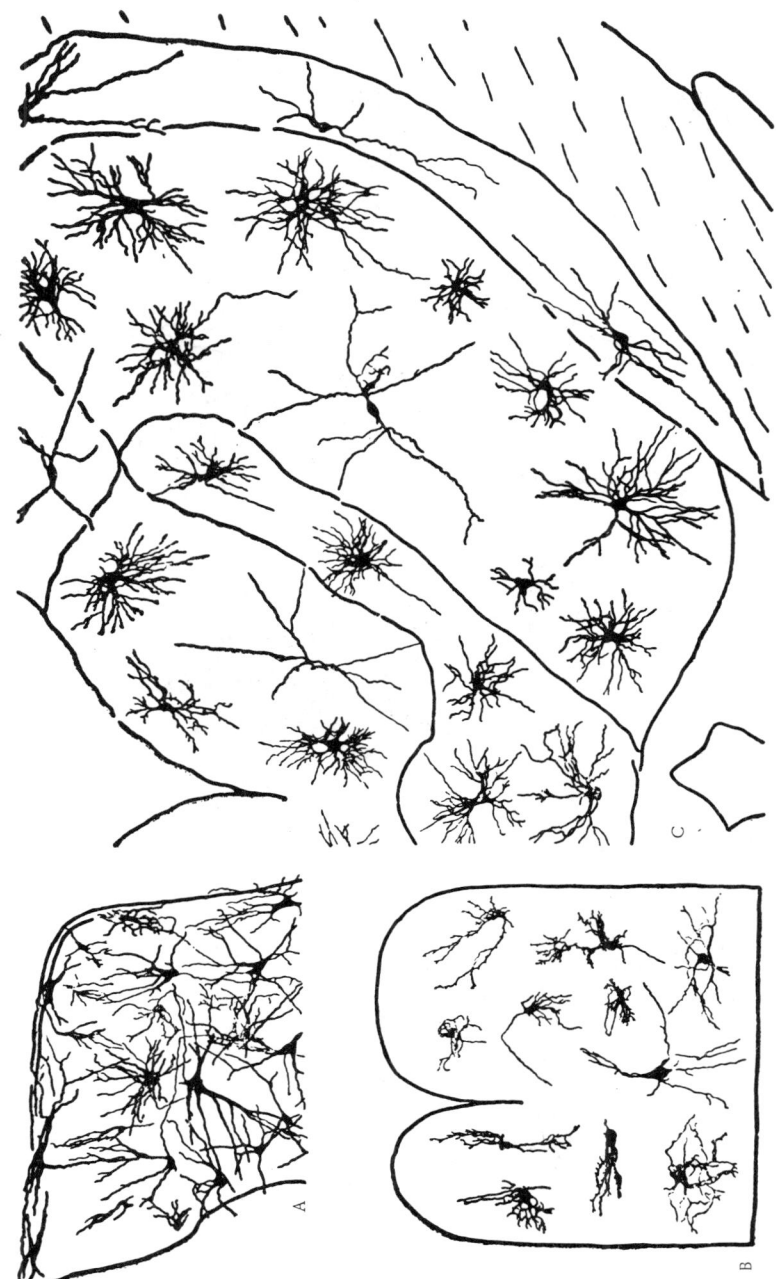

FIGURE 31. A — posterior horn of the spinal cord; B — transmitting neurons in nuclei of dermal and kinesthetic analyzers in the medulla oblongata; C — transmitting (relay) neurons in nuclei of the same analyzers in the optic thalamus (midbrain). Interspersed in the main mass of afferent multi-dendritic neurons are some neurons from the reticular formation, with few branchings (A and B after G. P. Zhukova, C — after T. A. Leontovich).

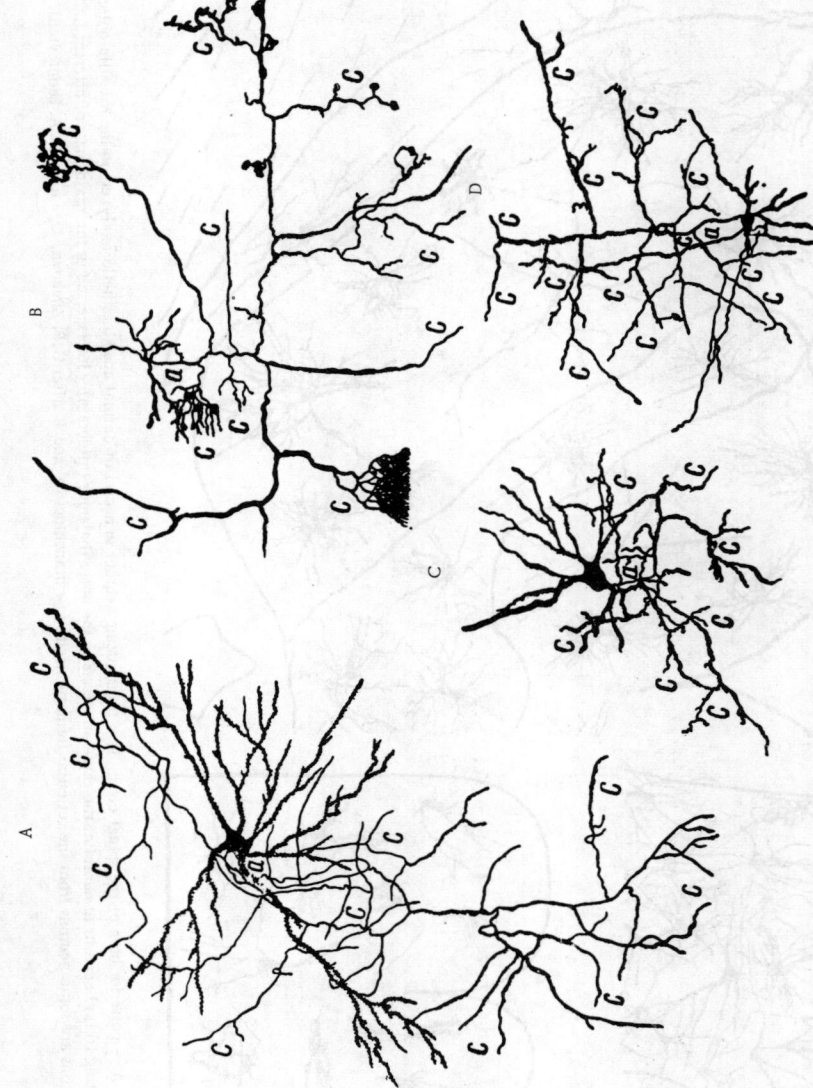

FIGURE 32. Various types of special transmitting (intercalated and intermediate) neurons:

A — reticular neuron in the posterior horn of the spinal cord (K. Gol'dzhi, 1894); B — reticular neuron in the medulla oblongata (M. and A. Scheibel, 1958); C — neuron with short axon from subcortical (basal) ganglia in the cerebral hemispheres (T. A. Leontovich, 1952); D — neuron with short axon in the cerebral cortex (G. I. Poliakov, 1956); a — axon of nerve cell; c — collaterals of axon.

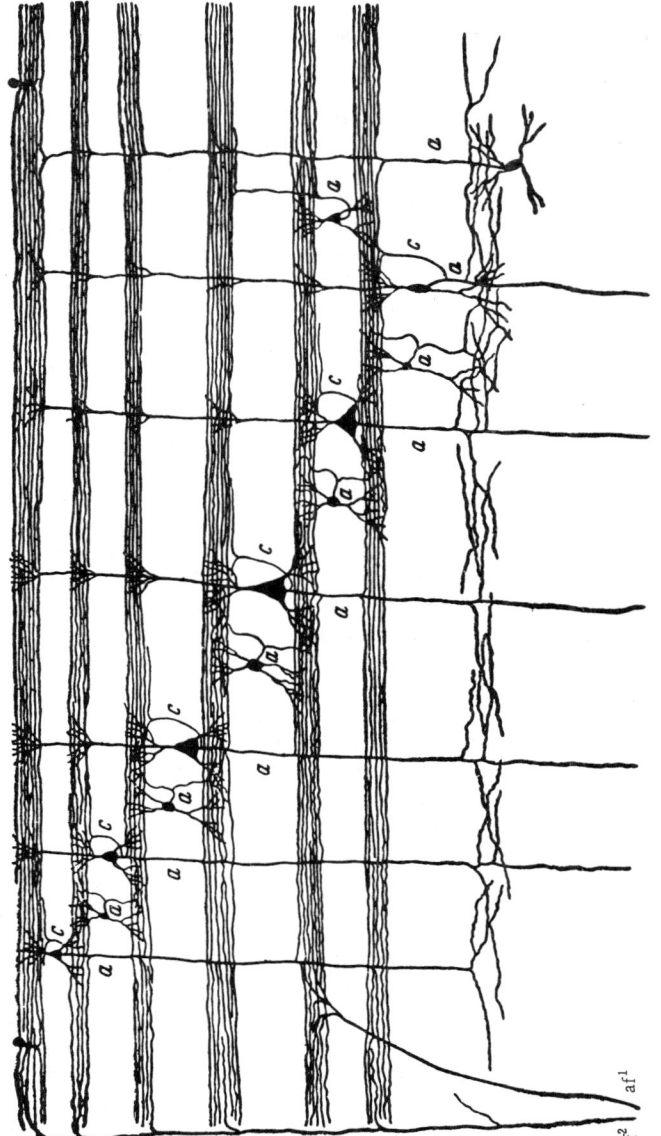

FIGURE 33. Diagram of networks formed by dendrite- and axon branches of nerve cells, horizontally orientated and penetrating the gray matter of the cerebral cortex. Depicted are pyramidal neurons with long descending axons and stellate short-axon neurons. Lateral and returning collaterals of long axons and branches of short axons are distributed in adjacent networks inside the cortex:

af^1 — afferent projected fiber passing impulses to the cortex from subcortical transmission stages of the analyzer systems;
af^2 — afferent associated fiber passing impulses from some points of the cortex to another specific point; a — axon of nerve cell; c — returning collateral of axon of a pyramidal cell (G.I. Poliakov, 1962).

both types contribute to the functional unity of efferent neurons, which with the terminal ramifications of their axons envelop certain groups of these neurons; together they participate in carrying out the various stages of reflex action (see Figure 14, rn; Figure 35, sl).

There are numerous short-axon neurons in the cortical sections of the analyzing-coordinating mechanism, for instance, in the cerebellar cortex and in the cortex of the superior corpus bigeminus, corresponding to the visual lobe of lower vertebrates and birds. Short-axon neurons are present in great numbers in the higher brain endings of the analyzer systems, forming the supra-axial part of the CNS, in subcortical (basal) ganglia of the cerebral hemispheres (Figure 32B) and especially in the cerebral cortex (stellate cells of the cortex, Figure 32D). Here such elements constitute a significance part of the highly differentiated network of dendritic and axonal ramifications of nerve cells which penetrate the cortical gray matter (Figure 33).

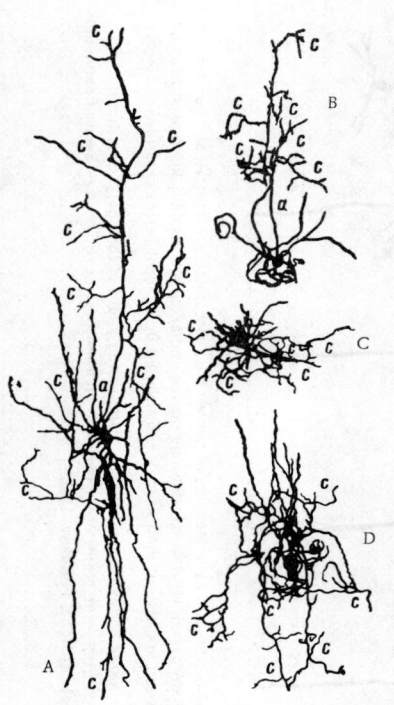

FIGURE 34. Different forms of stellate short-axon cells in the cerebral cortex:

A and B — stellate cells with ascending axon possessing numerous lateral branches; C — stellate cell with thin and fine axon ramifications distributed near the body of the cell, partially overlapping its dendritic branches; D — stellate cell the axon of which breaks up into a multitude of very thin and dense terminal ramifications oriented in different directions inside the gray matter of the cortex; a — axon; c — collaterals of axon (G. I. Poliakov, 1956 — 1961).

In the cerebral cortex, the ramifications of the short axons of stellate cells achieve a particularly high degree of fine differentiation (Figure 34); because of this structural pattern, a multitude of microscopic "combination centers" differentiate within the cortical gray matter (Figure 35) which may be assumed to represent the morphological basis of the mobile functional mosaic of stimulatory and inhibitory foci in the cortex described by Pavlov. The stellate long-axon cells, together with the main body of efferent neurons, are evidently the most important morphological structural components of the processes of analysis and synthesis of logical processes occurring in the cerebral cortex.

We have noted the structural differences between the reticular short-axon neurons conditioned by specific features of various interneuron connections. In addition to the indicated differences there are also certain similar features in the structures connecting the two types of element, which justify their inclusion in a single general group of special transmitting neurons. The facts substantiating this assumption are referable mainly to the particular nature of contacts, or synaptic associations, between the neurons (see following section).

The distinction of functional features of neurons, which we related to a single general group of special transmitting elements, has also been demonstrated by electrophysiological methods. Their specific feature, as mentioned before, is the capacity to generate rhythmic high-frequency discharges in response to a single stimulus — up to 1,000 impulses or more per second. Such a reaction is characteristic for particular reticular neurons in the axial part of the CNS (P. G. Kostyuk, 1962), and also for intermediate, short-axon neurons in the cerebral cortex. Functionally analogous elements were also detected in subcortical formations of the analyzer systems.

4. FORMS OF CONTACTS AND FUNCTIONAL INTERRELATIONS OF NEURONS

It is possible to distinguish two main forms of contact associations between neurons (synapses) in the CNS, which is characterized by a great variety of interneuron connections. The main means of interneuron connections are represented by the end terminal ramifications of axons, which approach the bodies and dendrites of other nerve cells and contact them by means of small terminal swellings of different forms (Figure 36, p, s, sl; Figure 37B, 1, 2). Such terminal synaptic apparatuses which, according to our observations, appear very early in embryonic life, are apparently adjusted for transfer of direct actions from certain neurons to others.

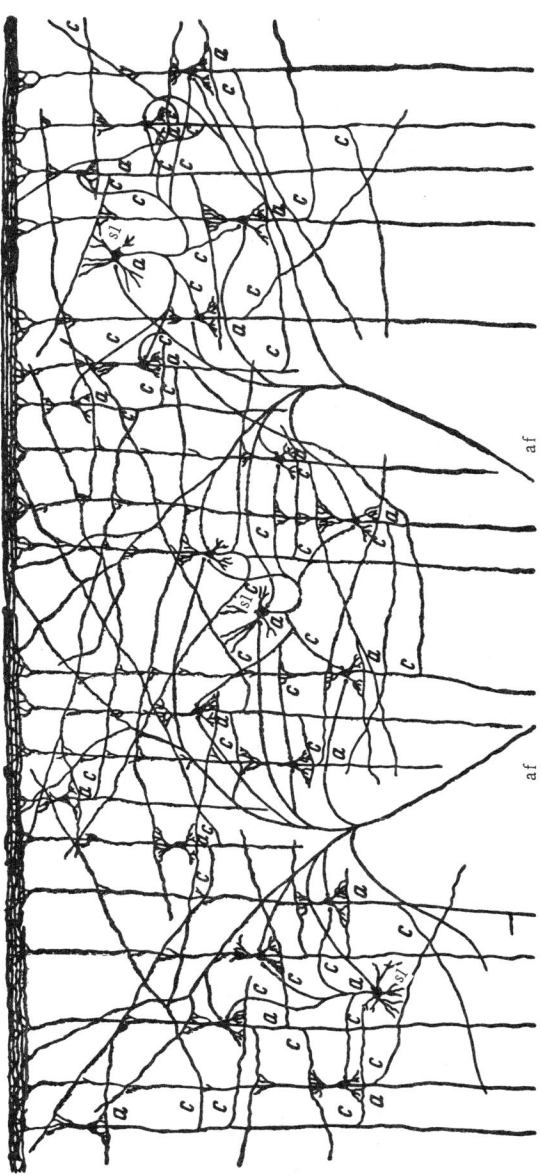

FIGURE 35. Elements of neuron structure constituting the anatomical basis for the multifunctional mosaic of the cerebral cortex. Depicted are centripetal afferent fibers (af) entering the cortex from subcortical sections of analyzers and forming numerous contacts with efferent neurons with long axons — pyramidal cells — as well as with special transmitting neurons — stellate, short-axon cortical cells (sl). Each stellate cell produces a functional union of a group of pyramidal cells and forms a microscopical "combination center"; a — axon; c — collateral ramifications of an axon (G.I. Poliakov, 1961).

Another type of formation of contact associations develops during later stages of ontogenesis, along with further development and differentiation of axonal terminal contact apparatuses in higher cerebral representations of analyzers, together with a progressive increase in the number of dendritic ramifications. This form of contact is realized through cytoplasmic dendritic processes on nerve cells, so-called lateral outgrowths ("spines") (Figure 37A, 1, 2, 3, 7). Dendritic processes with terminal swellings ("knobs") and the ends of axons both represent particular specialized synaptic formations. The knobs of the lateral outgrowths establish direct contacts with the approaching terminal branches of axons, as well as mainly tangential contacts with bypassing axonal ramifications and collaterals (Figure 37B, 3, 4, 5 and also Figure 36).* This form of contact, initially identified by us in specimens stained by the chrome-silver method, was also noted in electron microscope examinations by E. G. Gray.**

The main function of tangential contacts of axonal ramifications of lateral dendritic outgrowths is apparently the establishment of indirect tangential effects of some neurons on others; impulses addressed as terminal to certain neurons may incidentally, with the aid of contacts indicated, affect the functional condition of many other "extraneous" neurons.

The tangential contacts which which in ontogenesis (probably also in phylogenesis) appear later than the terminal ones may be considered as supplementary to the basic forms of interneuron connections in the CNS. The emergence of the apparatus of tangential contacts, supplementary to the terminal one, was evidently conditioned by further differentiation

---

* Contacts of axonal ramifications with lateral outgrowths on dendrites were first described by us in the human cerebral cortex in 1947. Later, they were also identified by co-workers at our laboratory (E.G. Shkol'nik-Yarros, T.A. Leontovich) in cortical and subcortical formations of various animals. The first reference to these contacts is found in the paper by E.G. Shkol'nik-Yarros. K istorii izucheniya tonkoi struktury kory mozga (History of Study of the Fine Structure of the Cerebral Cortex). — Zhurnal nevropatologii i psikhiatrii, Vol. 19, No. 1. 1950. We provided a detailed description of these formations together with an interpretation of their possible functional significance in a series of investigations (G.I. Poliakov. O tonkikh osobennostyakh struktury golovnogo mozga cheloveka i funktsional'nyk vzaimodeistviyakh mezhdu neironami (Details of the Finer Structure of the Human Brain and Functional Interrelations of Neurons). — Arkhiv anatomii, gistologii i embriologii, Vol. 30, No. 5. 1953; G.I. Poliakov. O strukturnykh mekhanizmakh mezhneironnykh svyazei v kore golovnogo mozga cheloveka (Structural Mechanisms of Interneuron Connections in the Cortex of the Human Brain). — Arkhiv Anatomii, Gistologii i Embriologii, Vol. 35, No. 2. 1955; G.I. Poliakov. O nekotorykh osobennostykh struktury neironov tsentral'noi nervnoi sistemy, obnaruzhivaemykh razlichnymi neirogistologicheskimi metodami. Soobshchenie 2. Kontaktnye apparaty, obrazovannye dendritami nervnykh kletok (Some Characteristics of the Structure of Neurons in the CNS, Detected by Various Neurohistological Methods. 2nd Report. Contact Apparatuses Formed by Dendrites of Nerve Cells). — Zhurnal nevropatologii i psikhiatrii, Vol. 61, No. 2. 1961; G.I. Poliakov. O strukturnykh mekhanizmakh funktsional'nykh sostoyanii neironov v kore mozga. Mezhdunarodnaya konferentsiya, posvyashchennaya 100−letiyu so dnya vykhoda v svet truda M.V. Sechenova "Refleksy golovnogo mozga," 24−30 noyabrya 1963. Tezisy dokladov (Structural Mechanisms of Functional Conditions of Neurons in the Cerebral Cortex. International Conference Dedicated to the Centenary of the Publication of the Work by I.M. Sechenov "Reflexes of the Brain," 24−30 November, 1963. Summaries of Reports). — Moskva, Izdatel'stvo AN SSSR. 1963.) In the recently published book of S.A. Sarkisov (Ocherki po strukture i funktsii mozga (Outlines of Structure and Function of the Brain). — Moskva, Medgiz. 1964.) two microphotos of our 1955 work are reproduced in Figures 61 and 92.

** E.G. Gray. Axo-somatic and Axo-dendritic Synapses of the Cerebral Cortex; an Electron Microscope Study. — Journ. Anat., 93, p. 4. 1959.

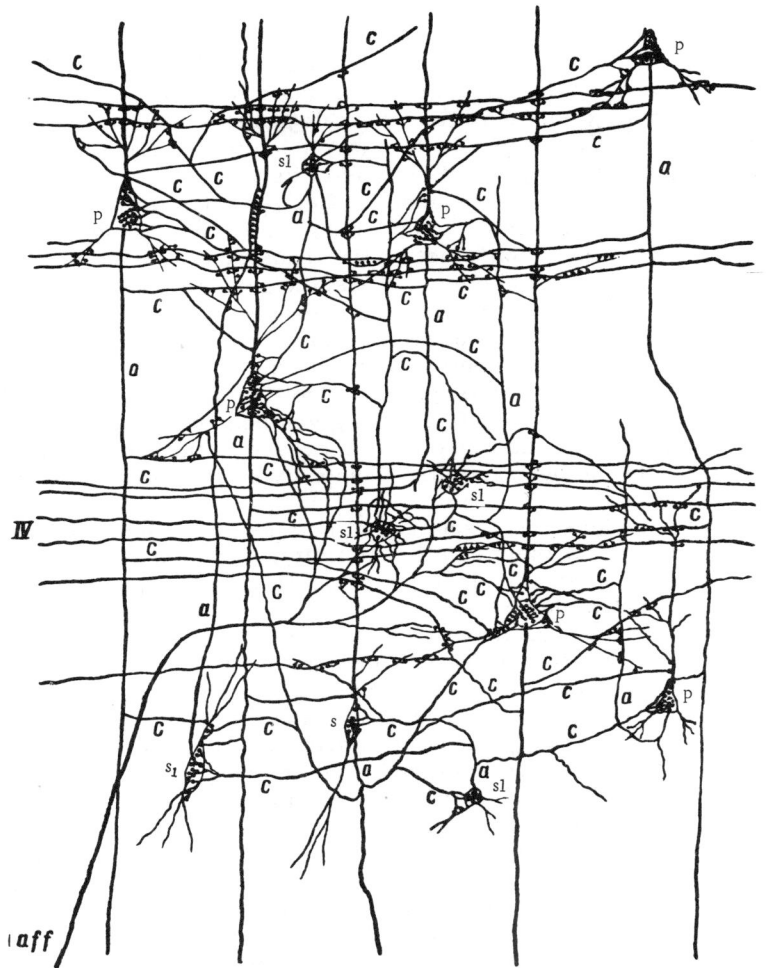

FIGURE 36. Forms of contacts serving different functions, synaptic links between neurons in the cerebral cortex:

aff — afferent fiber from subcortical areas of analyzer systems, their terminal ramifications forming contacts with both efferent and special transmitting cortical neurons; p — pyramidal cell with long axon; s — spindle cell with long axon; s_1 — spindle cell with ascending axon; sl — stellate cell with short axon; a and c — as in previous figure. The axon ramifications are seen to approach the bodies and dendrites of nerve cells, forming terminal synapses at points of contact. Note the "nests" or "baskets" surrounding the round cell formed by terminal ramifications of the short axons of the stellate cells on the bodies of pyramidal cells and other stellate cells. In addition to terminal contacts, one can see the tangential contacts, established by collaterals of axons with lateral outgrowths on the dendrites of nerve cells. These contacts are especially distinct along the course of the long horizontal nerve fibers (G. I. Poliakov, 1961).

during phylogenesis and ontogenesis of the entire structural pattern of axonal and dendritic ramifications in the most highly organized sections of the CNS.

The terminal and tangential contacts seem to have a different significance in neuron activity. The transfer of one basic functional state of the activated neuron to another (from a state of stimulation to a state of inhibition, and vice versa) apparently depends, to a large degree, on terminal contacts specialized for effecting direct actions of certain neurons on other neurons. On the other hand, indirect, tangential effects, realized by contacts of the tangential type, seem to have a supporting value only in the interaction of neurons, contributing or obstructing the transfer of a given neuron from one basic functional state to another. Thus, the general condition of each separate neuron at any moment of the execution of a reflex act is determined by the result of interactions of direct and tangential effects of many other neurons. In this case, evidently, the dendritic apparatus, which is the main effector of tangential contacts, plays the role of a finely adjusted modulator of the functional state as it affects the given neuron. With the development of dendritic ramifications there is an increase in the functional adjustability and reactivity of the neuron — its "responsiveness" to changes in conditions of other neurons.

In order to understand the nature of actions of some neurons on others during the process of their common activity, it is important to clarify the ratio of distribution of terminal and tangential contacts on the surface of the cell body and its dendrites in different neurons. We confirmed that the structure of dendritic distribution and number of lateral outgrowths are different in neurons with different functional patterns.

In cortical sections of the analyzing-coordinating mechanism (cerebellum), and particularly in the analyzer systems, the dendritic ramifications of efferent neurons with long axons are covered with numerous short, closely set lateral outgrowths; on the other hand, the body of the nerve cell itself and the first part of the dendritic outgrowth originating in it usually have two lateral outgrowths. In the cerebral cortex this type of elements are represented in the most typical form by pyramidal cells (Figure 37A, 1 and 2). A similar structure is also present in the long-axon efferent neurons of the most highly organized sections of the subcortical (basal) ganglia of the cerebral hemispheres (Figure 37A, 3).

Neurohistological studies have shown that the body of the cell deprived of lateral outgrowths, together with the first parts of the emerging dendrites, represent in the efferent neurons the main areas accessible to the terminal contact (synaptic) apparatuses. It may thus be assumed that the main functional condition (of stimulation or inhibition) of the efferent neuron is determined primarily by impulses acting on the central part of its entire receptor surface. On the other hand, the elaborate dendritic ramifications of the efferent neuron, which has a large number of lateral outgrowths, may be regarded as an additional receptor mechanism which exerts an indirect effect on its function. As a result, efferent cortical neurons are highly perceptive of a variety of impulses reaching the cortex from points closer to it or more remote, or impulses which circulate in various directions inside the gray matter.

Short-axon cells of cortical and subcortical ganglia (see Figure 32, B and D; Figure 34), specialized for other types of interneuron connections, are characterized either by the absence of lateral dendritic outgrowths (see Figure 34 A) or bear only single elongated lateral outgrowths (Figure 37 A, 5). Dendrites of reticular neurons of the brainstem (Figure 37A, 6) and spinal cord also have scattered elongated lateral outgrowths (Figure 37A, 7; see also Figure 30B) which thus indicate a certain similarity to short-axon cells of cortical and subcortical ganglia in the cerebral hemispheres. The presence of a similar aspect in the fine structure of neurons with short axons and in reticular neurons enabled us to relate both types to a single general group of special transmitting neurons, with certain functional similarities.

The physiological significance of these differences in the dendritic structure in efferent and special transmitting neurons (including reticular as well as short-axon cells in this group) is noted in the following: efferent neurons of the cerebral cortex and subcortical basal ganglia (as well as the cortical sections of the analyzing-coordinating mechanism distributed along the CNS axis) with their well-defined dendritic ramifications, supplied with numerous lateral outgrowths, evidently represent powerful impulse receptors, passing to them directly or tangentially (through tangential contacts with lateral outgrowths) and affecting their function. On the other hand, the special transmitting neurons, which include short-axon types or reticular neurons with a longer axon, possessing only a few dendritic outgrowths, or lacking them entirely, seem to be adapted mainly as points of contact for synapses, i.e., they function for the establishment of terminal contacts with other neurons. The elongated form characteristic for these elements, scattered in small numbers on dendrites of the lateral outgrowths, is evidently conditioned by the fact that special transmitting neurons, together with many terminal ones, form only single or relatively few contacts of the tangential type. This assumption is particularly relevant in connection with neurons of the reticular formation; it was possible to follow numerous terminal synapses extending their dendrites over a considerable distance (N. S. Kositsyn*). Judging from these structural features, the entire receptor surface of the short-axon cell as well as the reticular cell, may be compared with the central part of an efferent neuron. Elements of both types are evidently specialized mainly for convergence of impulses exerting a direct effect on their functional state. They themselves appear mainly as elements having a direct effect on other neurons.

This assumption is supported by our observations, which indicate that axons of stellate cortical cells and their terminal ramifications form extremely delicate networks appearing as "nests" or "baskets" on the bodies and on the first parts of dendrites of efferent neurons, pyramidal cells (Figure 36, p). From these data it is possible to conclude that the stellate cells are in a position to act directly on efferent neurons by uniting them functionally in a common activity. The sparse distribution of lateral outgrowths on dendrites of special transmitting neurons may indicate that those elements are apparently specialized for the formation of selective differentiated contacts with afferent and other neurons. The special transmitting neurons of various types which concentrate and distribute

---

* N. S. Kositsyn. Osobennosti akso-dendritnykh svyazei retikulyarnoi formatsii stvola mozga (Properties of Axo-dendritic Connections of the Reticular Formation of the Brainstem). — Doklady AN SSSR, Vol. 147, No. 2. 1962.

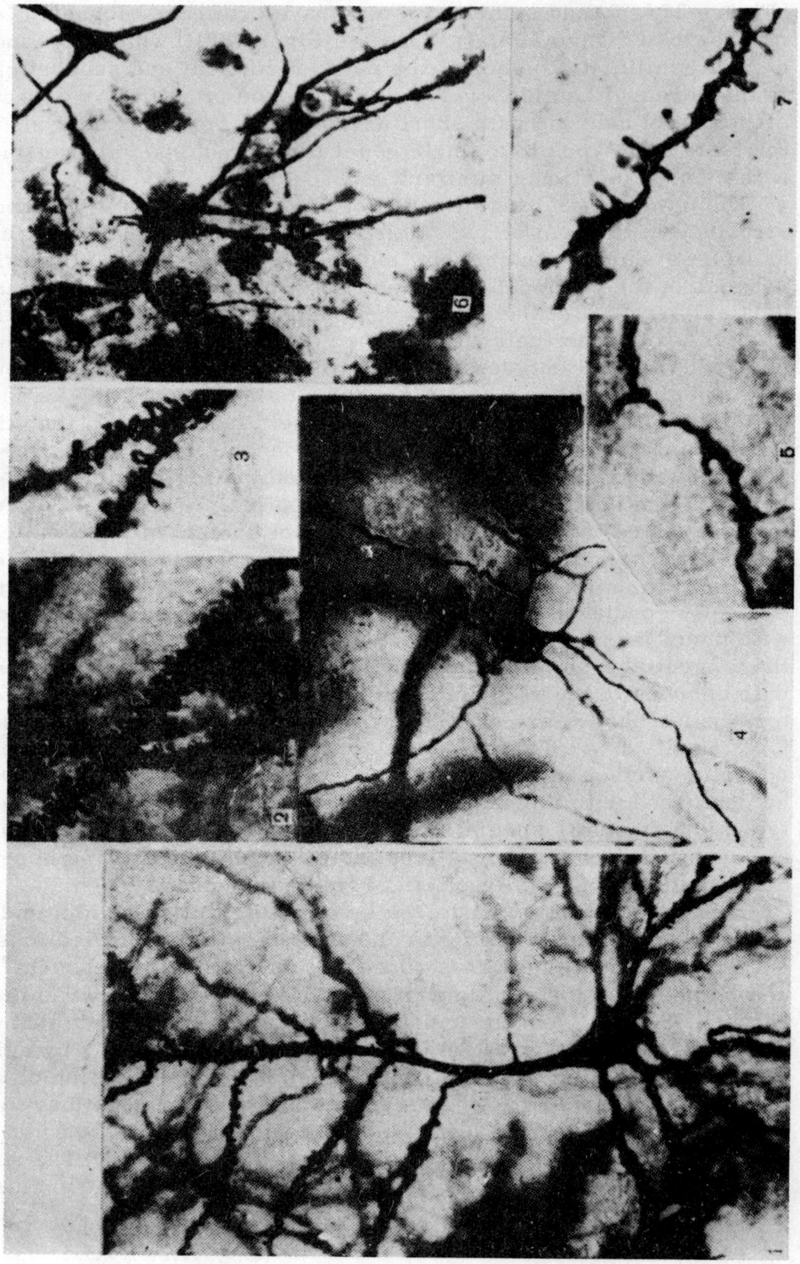

FIGURE 37 A

88

FIGURE 37A. Details of the fine dendritic structure of pyramidal and stellate cells of the cerebral cortex and reticular neurons. Photomicrograph of preparations:

1 – pyramidal cell; 2 – dendrites of pyramidal cells covered by numerous short lateral outgrowths; 3 – dendrites of an efferent cell with long axon, from subcortical ganglia, with a similar structure; 4 – stellate short-axon cell with smooth dendrites devoid of lateral outgrowths; 5 – dendrite of a stellate cell carrying sparse lateral outgrowths of elongated form; 6 – reticular neurons of the medulla oblongata; 7 – dendrite of a reticular neuron covered by sparse, very elongated lateral outgrowths (1, 2, 4, 5 – after G.I. Poliakov, 1953 – 1961; 6 – after G.P. Zhukova, 1959; 3, 7 – after T.A. Leontovich, 1959).

FIGURE 37B. 1 – terminal contact formations of axons on the body and first parts of dendrites of a pyramidal cell; 2 – the same on the body and dendrites of a stellate cell; 3, 4, 5 – tangential contacts (see x) of axons with lateral outgrowths on dendrites. Photomicrograph of preparations (1,2 – preparations by K.K. Blinova, 1961; 3, 4, 5 – after Poliakov, 1955).

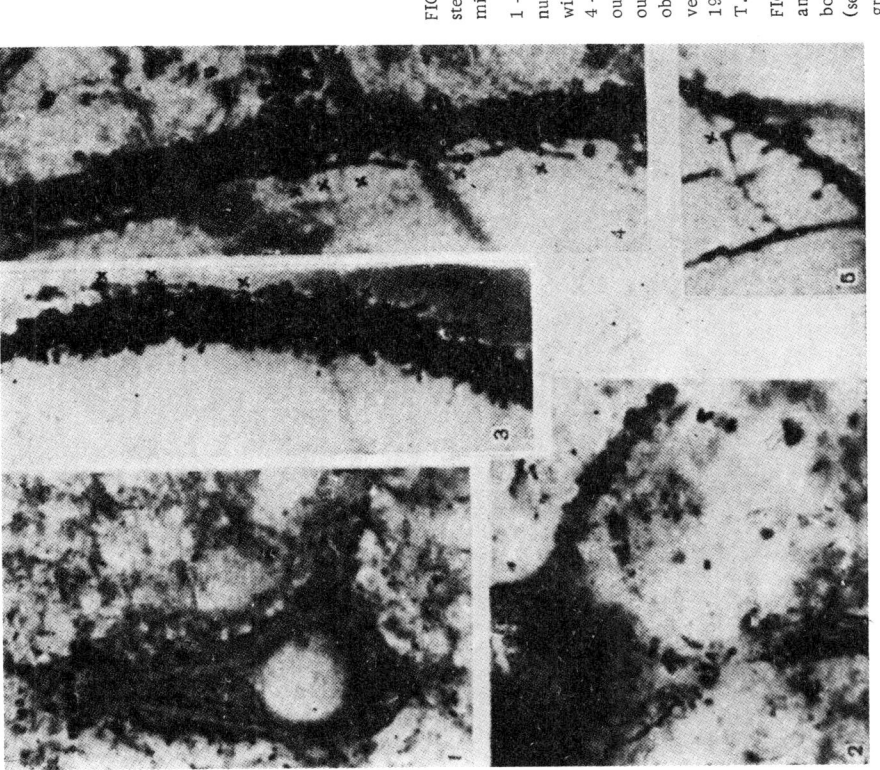

FIGURE 37B

direct effects are probably of considerable significance for determination of the functional condition (stimulation or inhibition) of efferent neurons.

The features of interneuron connections thus indicated, and established with the aid of special transmitting neurons, conform to our concepts of the special role of these elements in the processes of the delicate coordination of simultaneous or subsequent inclusion in the action of some groups of efferent neurons and exclusion of other groups.

Chapter IV

*THE BASIC PATTERN OF TRANSMISSIONS
IN THE NEURON NETWORK*

1. THE CENTRAL TRANSMITTING STRUCTURE
IN ANALYZERS

In the previous chapter we presented factual material and described some hypotheses concerning the origin and differentiation of neuronal patterns, as well as some elements included in the coordinating mechanism and in the analyzers. At the same time we noted the particularly important role of the special transmitting (intermediate or inserted) neurons in the structure of coordinating mechanisms and the analyzers. In this and subsequent sections we shall discuss in greater detail the organizational features of the neuron transmissions in analyzers, and we shall attempt to determine more exactly the role of special transmitting neurons in the entire system of neuron transmissions.

How are these elements formed and what are their topographic interrelations with other neurons?

In attempting to find an answer to this question, which is of importance for understanding the logic of the entire structure, we have again turned to the question of the origin of regulated reflex activity of the organism.

As already noted, it is typical that the course of a reflex act of any degree of complexity is coordinated. This is equally applicable to all stages in the execution of a reflex act. The clarification of neuron mechanisms ensuring the activity of analyzers, particularly of their most complex areas, is of cardinal significance in solving the problems raised previously in this connection.

When we first advanced the hypothesis on the origin of the neuron network (see Figure 27), we were able to devise a scheme explaining the formation of elementary coordinating structures. This scheme consists of a minimal number of interacting elements consisting of two receptor and two effector points (Figure 38A). In the presence of only one receptor and one effector, there is apparently no biological necessity of forming a special coordinating apparatus.

Figure 38B indicates that the elementary coordinating structure at the stage of development of a differentiated neuron network includes, in addition to lines of direct transmission of impulses from receptors to effectors, a prototype of a special transmitting neuron (n). This element, corresponding in a developed coordinating mechanism to a reticular neuron, is distributed in the central components of both reflex arcs (compare with Figure 10B, 3).

Turning to the question of the origin of the transmitting structure in analyzers, we proceed from our earlier assumption that in animal evolution the analyzers developed as a further differentiation of the functional possibilities inherent in the coordinating mechanism itself, from the moment of its formation. The reorganization of the system of transmissions and analyzers, compared with that of the coordinating mechanism (see Figure 10B), is interpreted by us as a multiplication of the elementary coordinating structure (elementary part of the coordinating mechanism) in connection with the tremendous differentiation of impulses transmitted through the analyzer.

We can present this process graphically if we represent the scheme of elementary coordinating mechanisms (see Figure 10B) such that the distribution of components will be oriented towards the same ascending direction (Figure 39A) to which the neurons in the ganglia of transmission in analyzers are oriented (Figure 39B). In this representation we can see that the special short-axon transmitting neurons are distributed in analyzers between the efferent long-axon neurons included in the parallel chains of impulse transmissions. The underlying similarity in distribution of these types of elements in analyzers and of special transmitting neurons of the reticular formation in the reflex arcs of the spinal cord and brainstem is confirmed.

The reorganization of the central transmitting structures in the analyzers as compared with the coordinating mechanism seems to be conditioned by the following factors. In the coordinating mechanisms this structure is formed directly between points of entry and exit of the CNS; in the analyzers it is "built in" in the chain of successive transmission of centripetal impulses from lower CNS levels. The formation of short-axon neurons in analyzers is one of the significant morphological indices of sensitive and complex differentiated processes of impulse transmission in the analyzing-coordinating mechanism, and especially in the analyzer systems. It seems that the special transmitting neurons of the analyzers, distributed in the zones of synaptic links of efferent neurons, play quite an important role in the processes of transformation ("logical reprocessing") of information and its "filtration," and this assists in the differentiation of significant impulses.

The further differentiation of the entire scheme of transmissions in analyzers was conditioned by the development of an apparatus of descending-centrifugal transmission, represented by the terminal ramifications of axons of neurons at higher levels, forming contacts with neurons at lower levels, along with the apparatus of ascending-centripetal transmissions of neuron impulses (Figure 39B).

One may assume that in analogy to interneuron connections in the elementary coordinating structure, there is also a principal scheme of convergence on efferent and special transmitting (short-axon) neurons of ascending and descending conductors in the analyzer (Figure 39B). The efferent and special transmitting neurons are included in the given transmission ganglia in the analyzer, under the constant effect of counterflowing distal or proximal impulses. It seems that the effect of the super structure and self-superstructure of analyzers on the action of stimuli, as a significant component of active concentration of attention on the investigated object, is carried out through this mechanism.

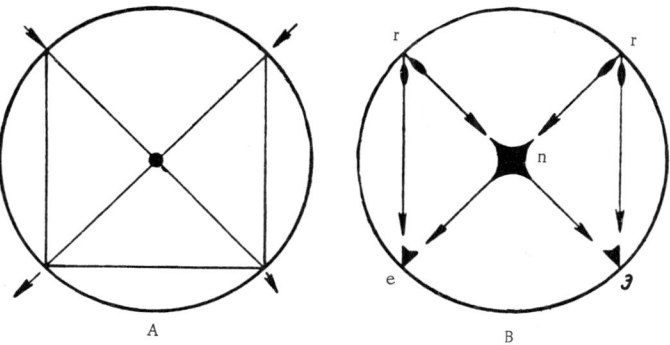

FIGURE 38. Diagram of the origin of the elementary coordinating structure:

A — the simplest combination of interconnections of two receptor and two effector points; B — elementary part of a neuron network consisting of two receptors (r), two effectors (e) and a special transmitting neuron (n).

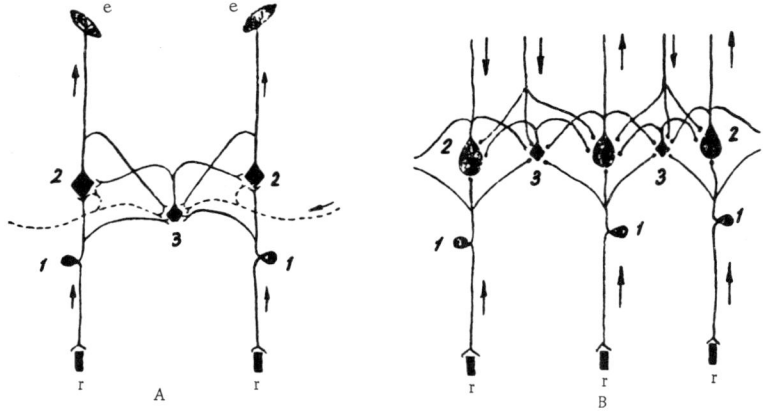

FIGURE 39. A. Transformed outline of elementary coordinating structure (compare with Figure 10 B) oriented in the same direction (see B) as the chains of neuron transmissions in analyzers. The markings and broken lines correspond to those of Figure 10 B.
B. Outline of structure of neuron transmissions in an analyzer (multiplication of the elementary coordinating structure): r — receptor; 1 — peripheral sensory neuron transmitting centripetal (afferent) impulses from receptors to efferent long-axon neurons (2) as well as to special transmitting short-axon neurons (3) included in the given corresponding ganglia. Ascending (centripetal) conductors (arrows pointing upward) are shown with descending (centrifugal) conductors (arrows pointing downward), corresponding to broken lines in outline A. As shown in outline B, the general plan of distribution of terminal ramifications into efferent and special transmitting neurons is uniform for centripetal and centrifugal connections.

We are still far from a clear understanding of the physiological nature of complex coordinating processes occurring in the cerebral parts of the analyzers and ensuring the adequacy of their reaction to external stimuli. It is evident, however, that these processes are based in principle on the same reciprocal interrelations of excitation and inhibition in functionally linked groups of neurons, as they exist in more elementary coordinating structures. A. A. Ukhtomskii emphasized that the reciprocal relations may involve the most diverse combinations (constellations) of neurons distributed in various sections of the CNS. Such a hypothesis explains some phenomena observed in delicate electrophysiological experiments (R. Jung*); in various links of analyzers at different moments of the action of stimuli, it was possible to detect certain groups of neurons reacting selectively (through excitation or inhibition) to inclusion, exclusion, or change in action of stimuli ("on" and "off" effects).

Our observations concerning the human cerebral cortex disclose that the special transmitting neurons (stellate short-axon cells) have a tendency to be distributed among groups of efferent long-axon neurons, such as the pyramidal cells (see Figure 35). This property of cortical organization may indicate that stellate short-axon cells unite groups of efferent neurons functionally, with the establishment of dynamic reciprocal relations; such a form of interconnnections between pyramidal and stellate cells corresponds to the topographic correlations between efferent and special transmitting neurons in the coordinating mechanism and in subcortical transmitting stations of analyzers, as indicated in our outlines (Figure 39 A and B).

We shall dwell briefly on our concept of the mechanism of the origin of special short-axon transmitting neurons in analyzers.

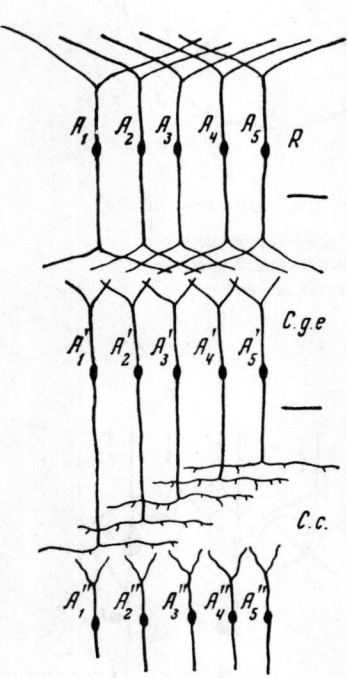

FIGURE 40. Outline according to Lorente de No (1934) showing partial interlacing of neuron outgrowths in transmitting stations of the visual analyzer system:

$A_1 - A_5$ – neurons of the retina of the eye (R); $A'_1 - A'_5$ – neurons of the subcortical transmitting ganglion (lateral geniculate body) (C. g. e.); $A''_1 - A''_5$ – neurons of the visual cortex (C. c.).

One of the fundamental structural features of analyzers is the principle of formulation, as a rule, of a partial interlacing of neurons (R. Lorente de No** (Figure 40)). Such a structure is characterized morphologically by the fact that in all transmitting formations of the CNS the terminal ramifications of the same afferent nervous fiber approach several efferent neurons at

---

* R. Jung. Excitation, Inhibition and Coordination of Cortical Neurons. – Exp. Cell. Research, Supp. 5. 1958.
** R. Lorente de No. Studies on the Structure of the Cerebral Cortex. II. Continuation of the Study of the Cornu Ammoni System. – Journ. f. Psycholog. und Neurol., Vol. 46, Nos. 2 and 3. 1934.

the same time. With this, the terminal ramifications of different nerve fibers interlace with each other. Thus a single efferent neuron establishes contact with several afferent fibers in the vicinity, i. e., is affected by impulses approaching it through different impulse conductors. This interlacing of nerve-fiber ramifications is already distinctly noted on the level of fusion of neurons with receptors. As A. A. Otelin's* recent observations have shown, certain receptor formations in the skin (Vater-Paccinian sensory corpuscles) usually receive the endings of several peripheral nerve fibers (polyaxon receptors, according to Otelin).

We consider this pattern of structural organization of transmissions as a particular derivative of the universal scheme of intersection of pathways, uniting all receptors with all effectors, as we already described (see Chapter III, Figure 27). In reality, and conclusive for Lorente de No's law, each neuron in the node of transmissions serves as a point of convergence and divergence of chains of impulses transferred along the neuron.

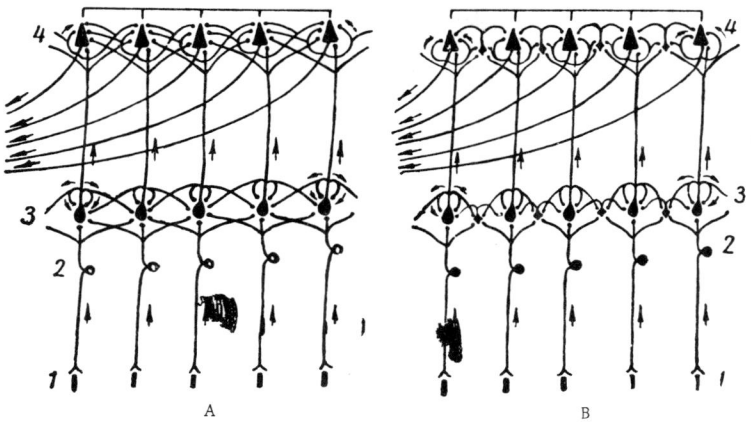

FIGURE 41. A. Outline of the transmitting structures in analyzers of a lower developmental level:

1 — receptors; 2 — peripheral sensory neurons; 3 — subcortical section of an analyzer; 4 — cortical section of an analyzer. Depicted are efferent long-axon neurons. The corresponding levels of this outline show only interlacings of terminal afferent fibers and recurrent collaterals of efferent long-axon neurons. In addition the diagram shows collaterals returning "on themselves" and approaching the body of the same nerve cell from which the axon of these collaterals originates.

B. More complicated outline (compare with A) of transmitting structures, corresponding to a higher developmental level of analyzers. Together with elements represented in outline A, the diagram also depicts special transmitting short-axon neurons formed at points of intersection of terminal ramifications and recurrent collaterals.

As shown in the diagram in Figure 41, the special short-axon transmitting neurons originate, in conformity with our concept (see Chapter III,

* A. A. Otelin. Nekotorye zakonomernosti razvitiya perifericheskogo kontsa kozhnogo analizatora v ontogeneze cheloveka (Some Patterns of Development of the Peripheral End of the Skin Analyzer in Human Ontogeny). — In: Struktura i funktsiya analizatorov cheloveka v ontogeneze. — Moskva, Medgiz. 1961.

Section 1) on the physiological mechanism of neuron origin, at points of crossing and intersection of impulse flows, transferred along the terminal ramifications of afferent fibers, and along recurrent collaterals of axons of efferent transmitting neurons (compare A and B in Figure 41).

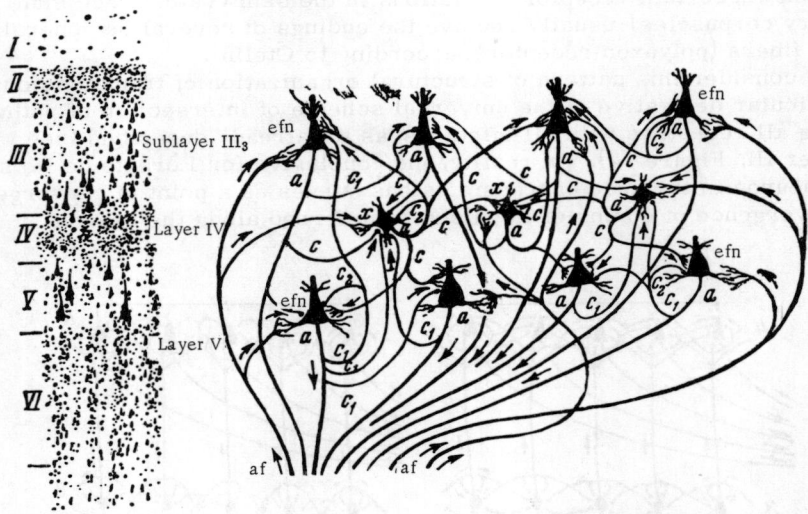

FIGURE 42. Partially schematic outline of interneuron connection in sublayer III_3, layer IV and layer V of the cerebral cortex. On the left are shown cytoarchitectonic layers of the cortex:

af — afferent fibers from subcortical transmitting stations of the analyzer systems; depicted are pyramidal long-axon cells (efn) of sublayer III_3 and layer IV, and also stellate short-axon cells (x) of layer IV; a — axons; c — collateral axons; c_1 — recurrent collateral axons of pyramidal cells; c_2 — collaterals returning "on themselves." Arrows show movement of nerve impulses participating in the completion of cycles of returning connections and interstimulations of neurons. For simplification of the scheme, only a few of the actually existing connections between afferent neurons, pyramidal cells and stellate cells of the cortex are depicted.

According to this concept it is possible to give a rational explanation of the origin of the inner granular layer of the cerebral cortex (Figure 42, layer IV). This cortical layer which plays quite a significant role in impulse transmission, entering the cortex from subcortical sections of analyzers, contains an accumulation of numerous so-called granulated cells of stellate and pyramidal form with short axons distributed at varying sites, or bending upward arclike. The ramifications of short axons of the various cells are closely interwoven and are often interlaced. At the same level of the cortex, in which collections of special short-axon transmitting neurons of layer IV are concentrated, there is a dense network of terminal ramifications of afferent fibers, also interlacing, entering from the subcortical formations of the brain. Our investigations indicate that these afferent fibers contact not only special transmitting stellate neurons but also long-axon efferent neurons in the pyramidal layer III (sublayer III$_3$) and layer V of the cortex (see Figure 36).

Understandably, the general pattern of transmitting structures as represented in Figure 41 is only a simplification which does not represent the entire complex nature of actual coordinations between afferent, efferent, and special transmitting neurons in the different CNS formations at various developmental stages of the individual and the species. Vertebrate evolution reveals the structural specialization of chains of neuron transmissions in various directions. Depending on the functional specializations of corresponding formations, this process is expressed in the particular development of some morphological features, while others regress in the course of time. According to observations of G. P. Zhukova, T. A. Leontovich and E. G. Shkol'nik-Yarros, the subcortical ganglia of transmissions in the analyzer systems (so-called relay nuclei) are adapted for the rapid transfer of specific stimuli from the periphery to the cortex, with a distinct localization, and are organized according to the principle of somatotopic projection, characterized in particular by a limited development of collaterals in long-axon efferent neurons. According to our observations, the collateral ramifications of the long-axon efferent neurons, together with the ramifications of special long-axon transmitting neurons, represent a particularly significant development in formations having a cortical pattern and specialized for realization of the most delicately differentiated and complexly integrated forms of reprocessing of transmission impulses. A similar structural feature is also found in the phylogenetically new sections of the subcortical ganglia of the cerebral hemispheres, which during ontogenesis and phylogenesis develop from the same formations of the cephalic vesicle as the fully developed cortical formations, and show a basic similarity to the latter in the particular details of their neuron structure.

2. CENTRAL NERVOUS APPARATUSES OF PERCEPTION AND IMPRESSION

One of the most characteristic features of the transmitting formations of analyzers is the creation of maximally favorable physiological conditions for the impression of actions of stimuli. As Figure 43 indicates, the interconnecting linkages of all transmitting elements are so constructed as to ensure (according to the theories of A. Forbes,* R. Lorente de No** and others, on completed cycles of interneuron connections) a continuing circulation of impulses at points of their transmission and a constantly renewed excitation of neurons, which interchange impulses with each other.

This mechanism provides for a continuous retention of stored traces of excitations in the process of their transmission through analyzers;

---

* A. Forbes. Interpretation of Spinal Reflexes in Terms of Present Knowledge of Nerve Conduction.— Physiol. Rev., Vol. 2. 1922.

** R. Lorente de No. Analysis of the Activity of Chains of Internuncial Neurons.— Journ. Neurophysiol., Vol. 1. 1937.

this was shown in contemporary neurophysiological studies which registered potentials passing outward from various points of impulse transmissions. Figure 43 A and B shows the anatomical-physiological mechanism of stored retention of traces of excitation including, as the most significant part, special short-axon transmitting neurons of the stellate type (in the most highly organized cerebral cortical formations most recently developed in the course of evolution) The stellate cells, included in the complex constellations of the efferent cortical neurons, acting together with subcortical mechanisms, apparently play an important role both in the function of impression of excitations reaching the cortex and in the processes of formation and reproduction of differentiated sensory activity and perception of objects in the external world.

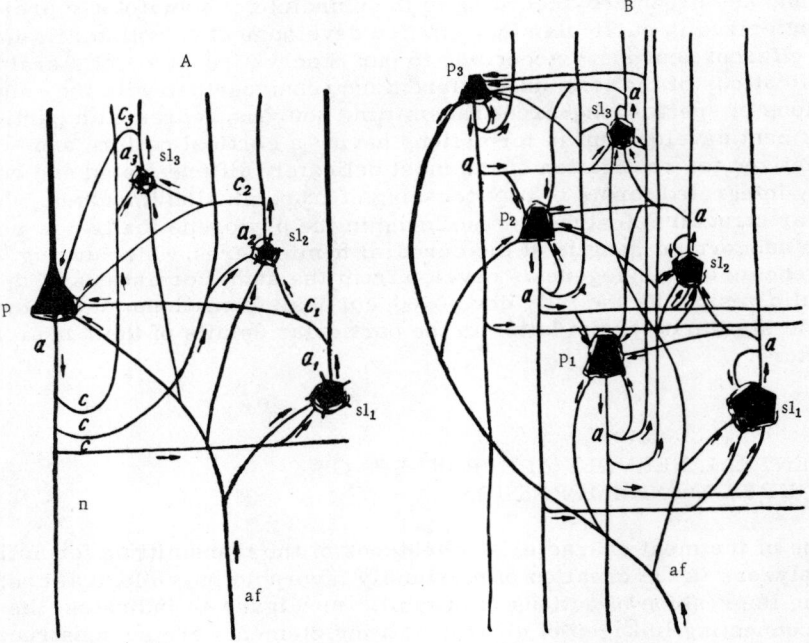

FIGURE 43. A. Scheme of interconnections between an afferent fiber (af), a pyramidal cell (p) and stellate cells (sl_1, sl_2, sl_3), which form the anatomical basis of continuous interconnections of impulses in the cerebral cortex:

a — long axon of a pyramidal cell; a_1, a_2, a_3 — short axons of stellate cells; c_1, c_2, c_3 — collaterals of axons. The arrows indicate the directions of continuous interconnections of nerve impulses inside the cortex, entering the cortex along the afferent fiber and leaving it along the long descending axon of an efferent neuron (n) (G. I. Poliakov, 1953).

B. More complicated (compared with A) scheme of continuous impulses in the cortex, illustrating in principle the same functional interconnections between an afferent (af) cell, pyramidal cells (p_1, p_2, p_3) and stellate cells (sl_1, sl_2, sl_3). Note returning axon collaterals, through which the neuron establishes contacts "with itself" (mechanism of self-stimulation of neurons) (G. I. Poliakov, 1953).

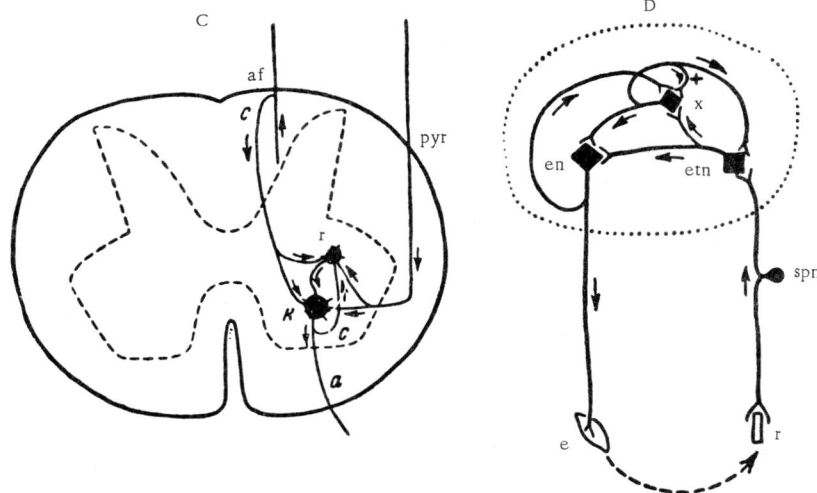

FIGURE 43. C. Diagram of continuous interconnections of impulses in reflex nerve centers of the spinal cord:

af — afferent fiber transferring centripetal impulses from receptors; pyr — fiber of pyramidal tract transferring centrifugal impulses from the cerebral cortex; k — effector (motor) neuron; r — special transmitting (reticular) neuron; a — axon; c — collateral of axon.

D. Revised diagram of a reflex arc. It indicates the position of the special transmitting neuron (x) in the reflex arc and the types of interconnections of the latter with the other neurons of the reflex arc. This diagram illustrates the special significance of this element in the completion of cycles of returning transmission and in the realization of continuous interconnections of acting impulses in the central part of the reflex arc during their entry into transmission centers from receptors (r) to effectors (e); spn — peripheral sensory neuron; etn — efferent transmitting neuron; en — effector neuron.

A further advance in the mechanism of interexcitation of neurons in the direction of an even finer functional differentiation is the formation of a special apparatus of self-excitation of separate neurons. The anatomical basis of this process is represented, according to our experimental results concerning the cerebral cortex, by returning axonal collaterals terminating in the body and dendrites of the same nerve cell (see Figure 41B, Figure 42, Figure 43B). I. S. Beritashvili* considers this structural detail of the cortical component of the analyzers and of the specially determined stellate cells of the cerebral cortex, with overlapping ramifications of their dendrites and axon, to be of special importance, and he defines such elements as cobweblike cells (see Figure 34C).

In order to understand the functional significance of stellate cells in the complex processes of perception, accumulation and impression of their traces in the brain, the experimental physiological study by

---

* I. S. Beritashvili. O strukturnykh i fiziologicheskikh osnovaniyakh psikhicheskoi deyatel'nosti (Structural and Physiological Basis of Mental Activity). — In: Gagrskie besedy, Vol. 4. Strukturnye i funktsional'nye osobennosti korkovykh neironov. Tbilisi. 1963.

N. S. Popova,* carried out in the laboratory of O. S. Adrianov, is of particular interest.

In this work Adrianov attempted to understand the mechanisms of movement and interaction of nervous processes, demonstrated by the method of conditioned reflexes, by comparing and noting the differences in neuron structure in the visual and auditory analyzers. On the basis of this analysis, the presence of a certain correlation between structure and function was deduced. The study clearly demonstrated a more prolonged persistence both of trace processes from conditioned stimuli and of the latent period, and less mobile nervous processes in the visual analyzer system as compared with that of the auditory one.

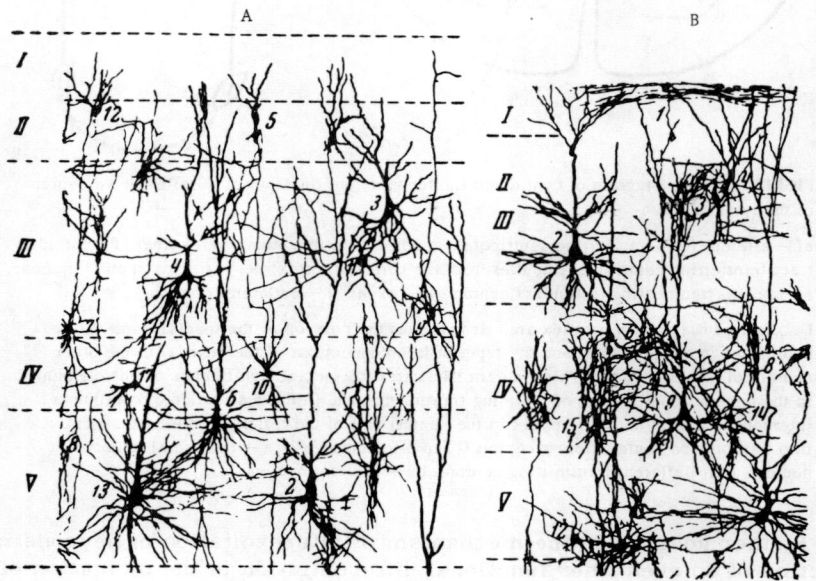

FIGURE 44. A. Neuron structure of the auditory field of the cerebral cortex in the dog (field T_3, according to the architectonic chart by O. S. Adrianov and T. A. Mering).

B. Neuron structure of the visual cerebral cortex in the dog (field O_1, according to the same chart). On the left are marked the layers of the cortex. When A and B are compared, it is seen that there are relatively few stellate cells in the auditory cortex (A, 7–11) and they have considerably fewer ramified outgrowths than the stellate cells of the visual cortex (B – 3, 6, 7, 8, 14, 15), the outgrowths of which form very thin and dense ramifications in the gray matter of the cortex. (A – after N. S. Popova, 1960; B – after E. G. Shkol'nik-Yarros, 1954.)

These physiological indexes are closely related to the histological features typifying the cortical endings of both analyzers, and especially with differences in structure and distribution of stellate cells in the visual and

---

* N. S. Popova. Sravnitel'naya kharakteristika dinamiki nervnykh protsessov v slukhovom i zritel'nom analizatorakh sobaki primenitel'no k osobennostyam ikh stroeniya (Comparative Characteristics of the Dynamics of Nervous Processes in the Auditory and Visual Analyzers of the Dog as Represented by Specific Structural Features). Candidate Thesis. Moskva. 1960.

auditory cortex (Figure 44). According to studies by E. G. Shkol'nik-Yarros (Figure 44B), the stellate cells are very densely placed, occur in large numbers and form thick and thin axonal networks. The short axons of stellate cells in the fields of the auditory cortex (Figure 44A) form considerably more diffuse and sparse ramifications, and the same cells are less frequent in the visual cortex. Thus, impulses in the visual cortex pass through a considerably greater number of transmissions than in the auditory cortex; correspondingly, conditions arise in the visual cortex which favor a more prolonged execution and persistence of nervous impulses.

The organizational features adapted to impressions of the diverse incoming external and internal impulses in the brain are apparently directly related to the main problem of orientation and reflex movement of the organism in space and time. Animals and man are able to perceive and react to events occurring around and inside themselves and they can also accumulate stored impressions of reality. The organism is also capable of not producing direct motor responses to stimuli, preserving traces of acting stimuli and reactions produced by those as images of memory of events in the past, and as a method of accumulating experience used in strategy and tactics of future behavior. The components of mental manifestations experienced by man are based on interacting chains of physiological processes occurring in corresponding structures of the cerebral cortex, and are related to complex space-time integrations realized in the cortex.

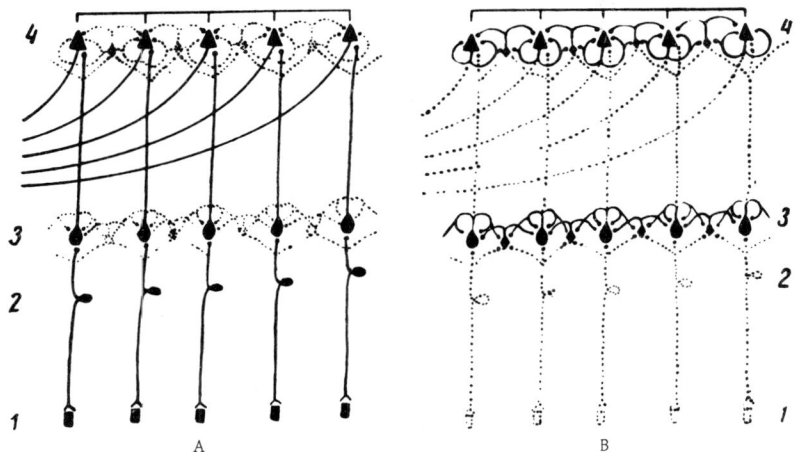

FIGURE 45. Diagram of two aspects of neuron structure indicating the morphological basis of reflex mechanisms of the organism effected by relations in terms of space (A) and time (B). Those elements of neuron structure which are of predominant significance in the corresponding form of reflex activity are depicted in black; the dotted line depicts those elements which play a supporting role in the activity of the conducting complexes of neurons. Explanation in the text.

Following the general scheme of neuron-transmission organization (see Figure 41B), a different specialization of certain elements of this scheme may be conjectured; this would enable the organism to effect a reflex image of events taking their course in space and time. One may distinguish special structural features adapted both to carrying out reactions of the organism directed to objects in the surroundings, and ensuring continuous mental activity at various levels of consciousness and time. The most suitable structure representing objects and manifestations is one consisting of chains of neuron transmissions oriented in the direction of analyzer transmission and providing a geometric connection between certain points of the sensory-receptor surface with corresponding points in the cortical end of the analyzer (Figure 45A). Such a structure in the brain is represented most clearly by a so-called precise somatotopic projection (see also Figure 55).

Processes of thought and retention in memory of a consecutive course of events in time are probably related to other features of the entire structure. Following current views on the most delicate structure of interneuron connections and transmitting stations of analyzers (see Figure 43), we have reason to consider that the main physical substrate of this process consists precisely of those groups of neurons which specialize in maintaining the continuous, subliminal circulation of nervous impulses in completed circuits of interneuron connections (Figure 45B). The initial scheme of the "lattice-pattern" of transmissions in the analyzer systems presented in Figure 41B may be considered as a prototype of the apparatus coordinating time and space factors of the external environment with the activity of the brain.

3. THE STRUCTURAL BASIS OF LOCALIZATION OF CEREBRAL CORTICAL FUNCTION

The nineteenth century physiologist Munk compared the cerebral cortex to a geographic map with numerous distinctly demarcated "provinces" corresponding exactly to the sense organs and motor apparatus of the body. The detailed separation of the cortex in the more highly developed mammals — into architectonically different areas, subareas, fields and subfields — is conditioned by the fact that the cortical representation of the various analyzer systems (as present in animals with a fully developed neocortex) presents an intricate complex composed of several sections differing in structure and functional significance. The system of each analyzer — visual, auditory, skin or kinesthetic — is represented in the cortex as a particular and distinct area (Figure 46 A and B; Figure 47 A and B) related to the most delicate analysis and most complex synthesis of stimuli perceived by the peripheral endings of the given analyzer. I. P. Pavlov termed these areas the nuclear zones of analyzers.

Pavlov's concept of nuclear zones of analyzers was confirmed by numerous morphological-physiological studies. In K. S. Lashley's* experiments, for instance, isolation of the visual zone of the cortex from all its connections with other cortical areas in the rat had no effect on animal behavior regulated by visual stimuli. In such experiments, monkeys did not lose their ability to distinguish colors, degrees of brightness or the shape of objects.

---

* The Neuropsychology of Lashley. "Selected Papers of K.S. Lashley." New York, Toronto, London. 1960.

Inside each nuclear zone, a series of different specialized cortical fields is differentiated; they are connected with the peripheral perceptor surface of the analyzer system by the corresponding sense organ, through a different number of transmissions in the proximal and more distal subcortex (see Figures 52 and 55).

In the course of mammalian evolution, special sections, the central fields of nuclear zones (Figures 46 and 47, fields 17, 41, 3, 4), have formed inside the special areas of the neocortex, which is first developed in these animals (visual, auditory, skin and kinesthetic sensation). Due to their structural and functional features, these fields are adapted to a maximal detailed differentiation and systematic grouping of single stimuli; in man they represent the physical substrate of finely differentiated sensory functions.

The cortical formations under discussion are connected with the sense organs through the least number of transmissions in the subcortical sections of the analyzer systems (see Figures 52 and 55). It is to be noted that these connections are formed mainly on the principle of exact spatial agreement of each point on the receptor surface with a certain point on the cortical surface (the above-mentioned precise somatotopic projection).

In primates these connections in the visual analyzer system connect the zone of most acute retinal vision (macula lutea) with the corresponding area of the central visual field. According to some findings, the number of fibers directed mainly towards the region of the occipital pole of the cerebral hemisphere constitutes more than half of all fibers converging from the subcortical relay-nucleus of the analyzer (lateral geniculate body) in the visual zone of the cortex.

In the ascending line of mammals there is an increasingly fractional differentiation of the central section of the analyzer systems according to the somatotopic principle, noted both in the cortical and in the subcortical stations of transmitting impulses. Thus, in the rabbit, there is not as yet a distinct topographic delineation of receptors entering from various parts of the body, inside the transmitting relay-nucleus of the optic thalamus. In the cat the differentiation inside the nucleus, according to the somatotopic pattern, is quite distinct (I. S. Robiner*). It appears even more clearly in primates, in connection with a significantly advanced structural-functional differentiation of the cortical zone of the analyzer.

Together with the central field in the nuclear zone of each analyzer, peripheral zones are differentiated (Figures 46 and 47, fields 18 and 19, 42 and 22, 1 and 2, 6 and 8) connected with the receptor surface through a large number of additional transmissions in the subcortical sections of the analyzer systems (see Figures 52 and 55).

Experiments and clinical experience of many years have indicated that these cortical formations realize more complexly conditioned forms of awareness of the outer world; with their aid, functions of perception, impression and coordination between more or less complex combinations of stimuli are carried out. Thus, following the removal of fields 18 and 19 in dogs, disturbances in fine differentiation of visual stimuli were recorded.

---

* I. S. Robiner. O lokalizatsii kozhnogo analizatora v kore i zritel'nom bugre krolika i koshki (Localization of Skin Analyzer in the Cortex and the Optic Thalamus in the Rabbit and Cat). — In: Razvitie tsentral'noi nervnoi sistemy. — Moskva, Medgiz. 1959.

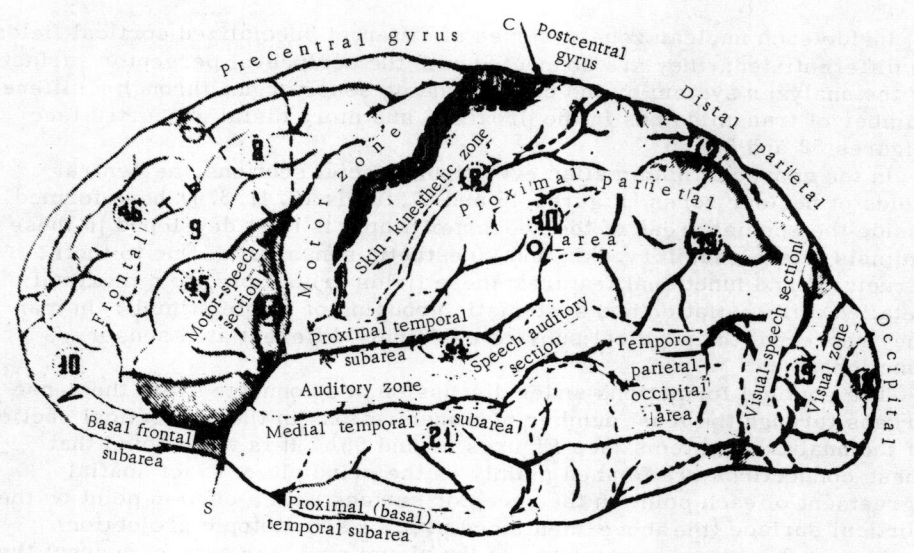

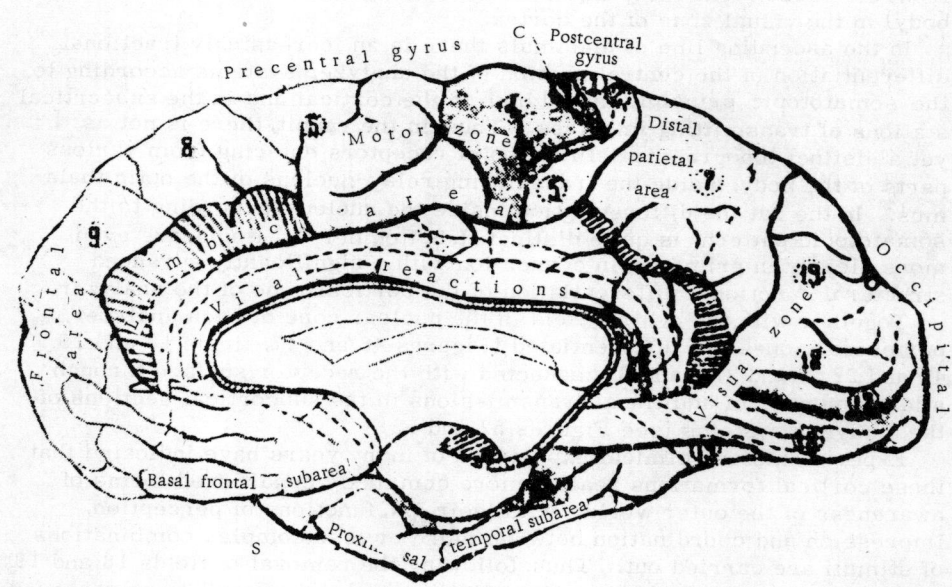

FIGURE 46. Charts of the distribution of cortical endings of analyzer systems and their corresponding cytoarchitectonic areas and fields on the surface of the cerebral hemispheres in man:

A — external surface of the cerebral hemisphere; B — inner surface of the cerebral hemisphere; C — central fissure; S — Sylvian fissure. The fields inside the areas are marked by numerals. Nuclear analyzers depicted: visual — in occipital area; auditory — in distal temporal subarea; skin-kinesthetic (sensory areas of body surface) — in postcentral gyrus; the motor zone of the cortex is represented in the precentral gyrus. The visual zone includes the central field 17 and the peripheral fields 18 and 19; the auditory zone — field 41 and fields 42 and 22; the skin-kinesthetic sensory endings — field 3 and fields 1 and 2; the motor zone — field 4 and fields 6 and 8; zones of overlapping of analyzers (internuclear zones) are represented by the distal (fields 5 and 7) and proximal (fields 40 and 39) parietal areas and by the medial temporal (field 21) and temporo-parietal-occipital (field 37) subareas; corresponding to them is the frontal area (fields 9, 46, 10). Distinct differentiation is found for the following sections: speech-motor (fields 44 and 45 of the proximal frontal convolution), speech-auditory (posterior section of field 22 of the distal temporal subarea) and visual-speech zones (adjacent parts of visual field 19 and proximal parietal field 39). The internal (limbic area) and proximal (basal frontal and basal temporal subareas) surfaces of the cerebral hemisphere, together with the insula near the Sylvian fissure, are occupied by the lower formations of the neocortex, and have a less differentiated functional significance. Together with the adjacent formations of the intermediate, old and paleocortex, these sections are related mainly to the olfactory and taste analyzer, to regulation of the conditions of the organism's internal environment and also to the vital reactions of the organism.

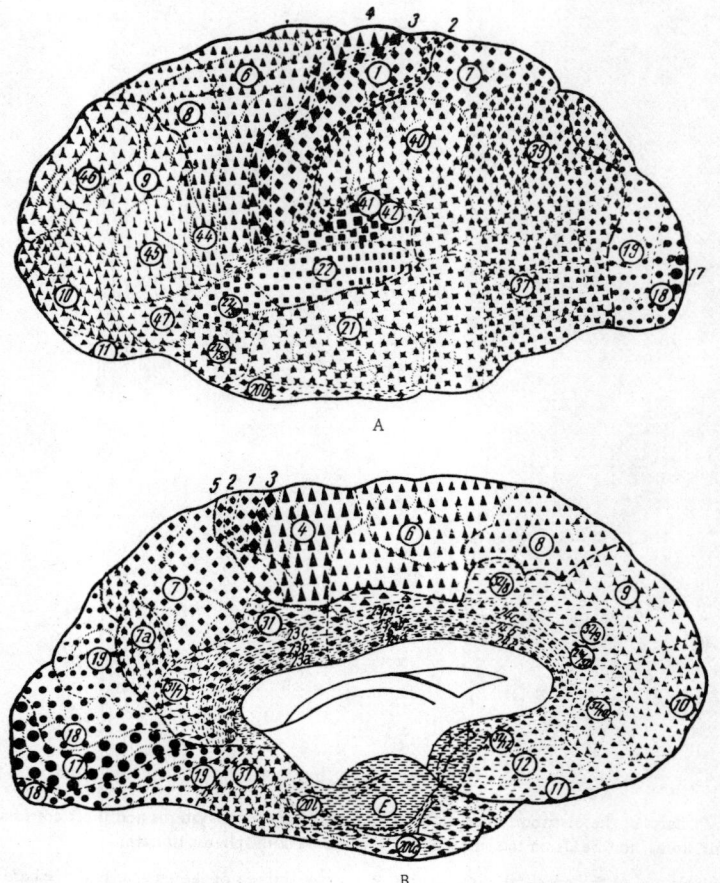

FIGURE 47. Diagram of topographic interrelationships among fields of nuclear zones and zones of overlapping cortical endings of analyzer systems on the external (A) and internal (B) surfaces of the cerebral hemispheres in the human brain. The numerical markings of the cytoarchitectonic fields are the same as in Figure 46. Each nuclear zone is depicted by a special sign in order to distinguish it from others: the visual zone by circles, the auditory by squares, the skin-kinesthetic (zone of body surface sensitivity) by rhomboids and the motor zone by triangles. The borders of the nuclear zones are marked by larger dotted lines, the borders of separate fields by smaller dotted lines. Inside each zone is the central field, marked by signs of the largest size, the nearest peripheral field by signs of medium size, fields in the peripheral zone by signs of the smallest size. The zone of overlapping of the visual, auditory and skin-kinesthetic analyzers (fields of proximal and distal parietal areas and temporo-parietal-occipital subareas) is depicted by a mixture of the signs of corresponding analyzers. The fields of the frontal area are represented by the same signs as the motor cortex, but these are more sparsely distributed. The speech-motor (fields 44 and 45) and speech-auditory (back part of field 22) sections are identified by a slightly different shape of signs selected for the corresponding nuclear zones. The marginal areas of the neocortex adjoining the formations of the intermediate, old and ancient cortex — the limbic area (fields 23, 24), and insula (enclosed by the Sylvian fissure) — and also the functionally related fields of the neocortex distributed over the lower and inner surfaces of the frontal and temporal lobes of the hemispheres (fields 47, 11, 12, 20) are marked horizontally by closely set signs, alternated with horizontal strokes; the density of the latter increases as they approach the formations of the intermediate, old and ancient cortex (according to the classification of I.N. Filimonov) which are marked by coarser horizontal strokes (G.I. Poliakov, 1961).

The animals did not discern objects of slightly different shape; for instance, they would not distinguish between an octagon and a circle (M. M. Khananashvili*). In similar damages of the brain in monkeys other investigators have noted transitory disturbances in the acuity of vision, depth of perception, distinction between colors, shapes, size of objects, or direction of movement (L. V. Koroleva**). In man, excitation of fields 18 and 19 results in a more complex visual perception than following excitation of field 17, in the form of intelligent and definable images: colored rings, balls, figures of animals, faces, etc. In their studies A. R. Lurie and co-workers have shown in particular, that the function of simultaneous perception and retention in consciousness of the many separate details of a perceived object is related to a great extent to the peripheral components of the nuclear zone of the visual analyzer, and this aids in the integration of the total image obtained.

An example of complex physiological syntheses carried out in the cortical zone of the visual analyzer may be provided by the following observation. In the psychological experiments of Ames†, the subject was directed to look into the opening of a box where he saw a toy chair suspended in space. Actually, in different places inside the box separate points of this object were suspended by wires; in a certain direction of the experimental subject's vision they were perceived as an entire object. This illusory impression was preserved in the subject even when he had an opportunity to be convinced by direct visual control experiments that the separate parts of the suspended object were removed from one another in space.

There are reasons to assume that in the peripheral fields of the nuclear zones, topographic correlations exist between points of the sensory perceptor and cortical surfaces of a more complex type than in the central fields (see Figure 49). The principle of precise somatotopic projection is not particularly evident in the peripheral fields of certain analyzer systems, in distinction to all central fields. With all the specific features of their structural organization, the peripheral fields of the nuclear zones are adapted mainly to ensure various functional connections between the separate impulse stimuli, both within the limits of the same nuclear zone and the complex of nuclear zones related to different analyzers.

In the process of evolution, the topographic relations between cortical representations of different analyzer systems become more differentiated, together with the reconstruction of their functional interrelations, conditioned by the more complex environmental effects on the organism. Together with the more detailed structural differentiation of the central and peripheral fields within the nuclear zones (see Figures 24 and 48), a territorial expansion of cortical zones of different analyzers takes place, with

---

* M. M. Khananashvili. Eksperimental'noe issledovanie tsentral'nykh mekhanizmov zritel'noi funktsii (Experimental Study of Central Mechanisms of Visual Function).— Leningrad, Medgiz. 1962.

** L. V. Koroleva. Strukturno-funktsional'nye izmeneniya zritel'nogo analizatora posle udaleniya zatylochnykh dolei golovnogo mozga u obez'yan raznogo vozrasta (Structural-functional Changes in the Visual Analyzer following Removal of the Occipital Lobes of the Brain in Monkeys of Different Age). Candidate Thesis. Moskva. 1963.

† A. Ames. Visual Perception.— Psychol. Monograph, No. 324. 1951; A. Ames and N. H. Ittelson. The Ames Demonstrations in Perception.— Princeton Univ. Press. 1952.

increasing interconnections and the formation of overlapping zones of cortical analyzer endings.

The overlapping zones (they may be termed the internuclear zones of the cortex) are distinctly represented in primates by anatomically adapted cortical formations (note the areas marked by small dotted lines in Figure 24). To those are related the distal parietal (fields 5 and 7) and proximal parietal (fields 39 and 40) and the medial temporal (field 21) and temporo-parietal-occipital (field 37) subareas (see also Figures 46 and 47). The same group of cortical fields may also include, in accordance with their functional significance and their position in the line of other fields, certain fields (9, 46, 10) of the frontal area which, as already mentioned, represents nearly one-fourth of the entire volume of the cerebral cortex.

The neurons of the cortical formations under discussion are apparently connected with the sense- and motor organs in the periphery in a most complexly conditioned manner through a very large number of additional transmissions in the subcortical sections and cortex (see Figures 52 and 55). This may be determined physiologically in view of the fact that excitations of the peripheral endings of the analyzer systems, causing certain changes in the functional states of neurons of central and peripheral fields of nuclear zones, are not clearly discernible in the activity of neuron complexes included in the overlapping zones.

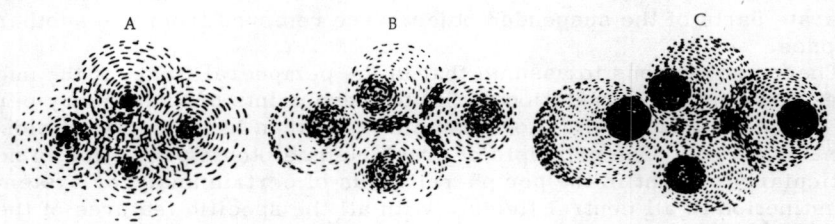

FIGURE 48. Diagrams depicting consecutive steps in the progressive differentiation of fields of nuclear zones and overlapping zones of cortical endings of analyzer systems in mammalian evolution. The increasing concentration of central fields are shown (marked by dark circles in diagram C) with an increasingly sharp delineation from peripheral fields of nuclear zones (marked by less closely drawn strokes in diagram C), with interference and formation of overlapping areas (marked by more closely drawn overlapping strokes in diagram C).
A — lower level of differentiation, in which the cortical zones of the analyzers are very "diffuse" and only partly separated from each other; diagram A corresponds to the level of development of the neocortex in Insectivora;
B — higher degree of differentiation, with distinct delineation of cortical zones, and inside those of central fields (closely drawn strokes) the overlapping of zones (marked by more closely drawn overlapping strokes) is still indistinct; diagram B corresponds to the developmental level of the neocortex in rodents;
C — still higher stage in differentiation with distinct separation of field groups within the limits of nuclear zones as well as zones of overlapping; diagram C corresponds to the developmental level of the neocortex in the lower primates (G.I. Poliakov, 1958).

These comparative-anatomical and clinical studies indicate definitely that the formations producing the overlapping zones are related to the patterns of human perception and action; they show a particular correlation to actual impulse stimuli (cerebral mechanism of speech, physical activity, creative imagination, thought, experience and foresight). These zones apparently represent the most important integral part of logical functions and representations of the most complex systems of relations between stimuli to the external environment, and appear as the physical substrate of processes of comparison, confrontation of objects according to significant factors denoting their similarities or differences (analysis and synthesis, classification), judgment, mental deductions, etc.

These briefly depicted differences in the functional significance of the different fields, conditioned by the specific features of the structure of connections and included in the cortical zones and overlapping zones of analyzers, were demonstrated more clearly in clinical and pathomorphological studies of N. S. Preobrazhenskaya.* In craniocerebral injuries three distinctly delineated clinical syndromes were differentiated, depending on the localization of the traumatic focus in the visual and adjacent cortical areas. Damage to the central visual field with its connections was usually followed by more or less distinct disturbances in perception of visual excitations; in cases of considerable damage to this area, cortical blindness occurred. In damage to the peripheral fields of the cortical zone with their connections, the clinical features first included disturbances in the function of visual perception and interpretation. In those cases when the site of damage included the cortical fields of the proximal parietal area and the temporo-parietal-occipital subarea, distributed in the vicinity of the visual zone, disorders of still more complex forms of cortical integrations appeared, conditioned by the interaction of visual and other analyzers. In such cases disturbances were observed in synthesis, orientation in space and reading and writing. According to clinical observations, there is a connection between the parietal area which, as mentioned, may be related to the overlapping zones of cortical endings of analyzers, and the formation of a concept of the general scheme of the body and of spatial coordination of its parts. Injuries to this area cause disturbances in posture and disorders of localization of direction of movement and position of different parts of the body.

4. GENERAL SCHEME OF INTERCONNECTIONS BETWEEN VARIOUS LEVELS OF TRANSMISSIONS IN ANALYZERS

In Chapter III, Section I a range of questions related to the problem of the origin of the neuron network was discussed. It was suggested that neuron structure is based on the principle of a universal crossing over of interconnections of all elements taking part in transmission and transformation of nerve signalling (see Figure 27). We have noted further that the same principle which expresses the most general features of brain structure also applies to the mechanism of the central transmitting structure in analyzers, the details of which we discussed in previous sections

---

* N. S. Preobrazhenskaya. K voprosu o narushenii vzaimootnosheniya pervoi i vtoroi signal'noi sistemy pri povrezhdenii mozgovogo kontsa zritel'nogo analizatora (Problem of Breakdown of the Interrelations of the First and Second Signalling System in Injuries of the Cerebral Endings of the Visual Analyzer). — Zhurnal Nevropatologii i Psikhiatrii, Vol. 52, No. 4. 1952.

of this chapter. We assume that the very concept of the structure of interconnections on the "grid" pattern serves as the starting point which may eventually lead to a rational interpretation of complex regularities determining the structural differentiation of the cortical endings of the analyzer systems, and the nature of their connections with each other and the subcortical areas (formation of the more proximal and more distal subcortex).

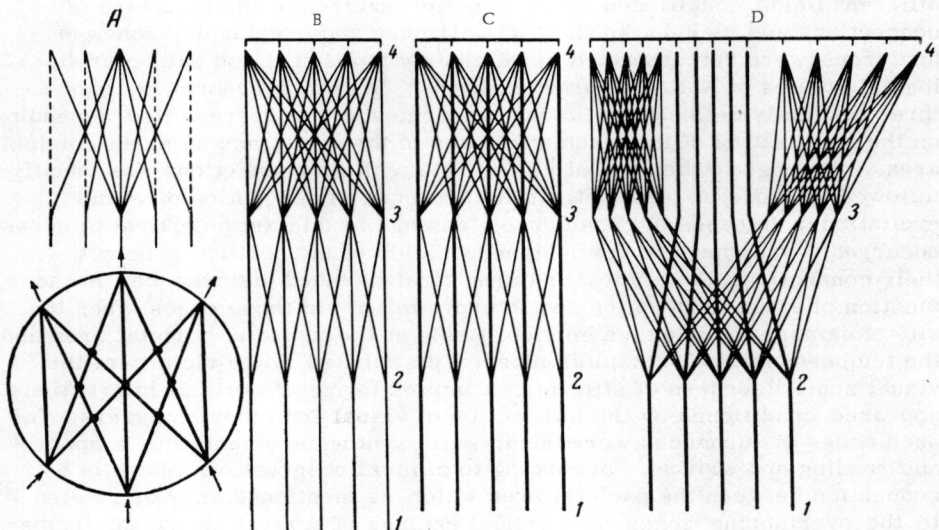

FIGURE 49. Diagrams illustrating the progressive differentiation, in mammalian phylogenesis, of the basic structure — the "grid" of interconnections at all levels of transmission along the analyzer systems:

A. Upper part, diagram showing the potential connection of each point of a lower level of transmission with each point at a higher level of transmission, and vice versa. Lower part, for comparison, shows a diagram of the origin of the elementary neuron network, oriented in the same direction (compare with Figure 27A).

B. Diagram of the "grid" in a mammal with low organizational differentiation of the brain: 1 — level of receptors; 2 — level of transmissions in lower (axial) parts of the CNS (level of distal subcortex); 3 — level of transmissions in proximal subcortex; 4 — level of transmissions in cerebral cortex (same markings as in other diagrams). The "grid" of interconnections at all levels of transmission retains its uniform character along the entire course depicted.

C. Diagram of the "grid" of a mammal with higher differentiation of brain organization. Inside the "grid" (marked by thicker lines) direct projections are separated through all levels of transmissions at certain points of the receptor surface to certain points at the cortical surface.

D. Diagram depicting a further step in the progressive differentiation of the "grid" interconnections. Individualization of the central field, in the cortical zone of the analyzer system, in which direct projections are precisely concentrated, and of peripheral fields which contain mainly indirect crossing-over connections between points of the receptor and cortical surfaces.

Following this hypothesis, it is possible to draw geometric diagrams (Figure 49) representing both an exact projection of certain points of the receptor surface at their corresponding points of the higher cerebral (cortical) endings of the analyzer system and an indirect, crossing-over connection of a particular stimulus receptor with another corresponding terminal point of the analyzer system.* This system provides the necessary conditions for the correlation of all types of combinations of stimuli; this enables the analyzer systems to be a universal apparatus which registers correctly any changes in the external environment, and provides a comprehensive method for interpreting their signalling significance for the organism. The schemes of interconnections represented in Figure 49 can also be useful for understanding the functional lability of the brain and the intersubstitution of its various components, clearly expressed in manifestations of compensation and partial recovery of lost functions in local brain injuries. These schemes are also of interest for clarifying the problem of reliability of the complex system represented by the brain.

We consider the progressive differentiation of the analyzer system in mammalian evolution to be a process of separation of various forms of organization of transmissions, connecting the receptor and cortical surfaces of the analyzer systems (Figure 49 C and D) out of the initial relatively uniform "grid" of interconnections between levels (Figure 49 B). On the one hand, there is a progressive powerful development and concentration of transmissions and pathways in the core of the entire analyzer system; through this the most direct, "precise" projections of the receptor periphery to the central field of the cortical zone of analyzers is established. On the other hand, parallel and interconnected with this process, are individualized collections of transmitting neurons and conductors, more and more specialized to form networks of indirect, crossing-over connections between points of the receptor surface and points of peripheral fields of the cortical zone of the analyzer.

Such a concept of brain structure conforms to results obtained in experimental stimulations or extirpations of central as well as peripheral fields of analyzer zones. This structure may in particular explain the detailed localization of projections of separate groups of receptors in the central fields, in the presence of a complex, intricately grouped representation of elements of the receptor surface and the peripheral fields, organized according to the principle of geometric conformity.

The diagrams in Figure 49 also provide an explanation for one of the most significant differences in the structure of the cortical components of analyzer systems and the analyzing-coordinating mechanism. The cerebellar cortex which, from specific features of its structure, may be regarded

---

* There is a striking similarity between our diagram of a universal "grid" of interconnections, on which the organization of the entire system of neuron transmissions in the brain is based, and the diagram illustrating the determination of an optimal variant of a solution to a problem by the mathematical method of sequential analysis, as worked out by V. S. Mikhalevich and N. Z. Shor. To prove this point it is sufficient to compare our Figure 49 with the diagrams presented in Figure 50, taken from a paper by A. Kondratov published in the journal "Nauka i Zhizn'," No. 11, 1961. Another example of this theory is the diagram in Figure 51 concerning the principle of action of perception, borrowed by us from the booklet by L. P. Kraizmer ("Bionika." — Moskva-Leningrad, Gosenergoizdat. 1962).

One may conclude from these examples that the most significant function realized by the complex analyzer system and well expressed in its structure also represents a "search," in an organization permitting a multitude of possible variants, for the most suitable solution of a biological problem; this is carried out with the aid of a sequential multistage analysis and synthesis of impulses transferred according to the transmission system in the analyzer.

as a prototype of the cerebral cortex, typically differs from the latter in its uniformity, homogeneity and "monotony" of structure. In the cerebellum the cortical structure pattern apparently does not attain the same degree of morphophysiological differentiation, in which separation of areas and fields specialized in a different manner according to structure and function takes place. This type of structure is, in turn, conditioned by the fact that the cerebellar cortex, in contrast to the cerebral cortex, functions as if on a single plane, i.e., it carries out in toto a uniform function of analysis and synthesis of one single complex of stimuli. This is correlated with the activity of the entire transmitting system connecting the cerebellar cortex with the receptor surfaces of the organism projected to it; this system is already formed at a stage when the grid of interconnections between different levels of transmissions still retains a relatively little differentiated, uniform character (Figure 49B). Only with the development of the analyzer systems does the organization of interconnections between all levels of transmission attain higher degrees of differentiation (Figure 49 C and D).

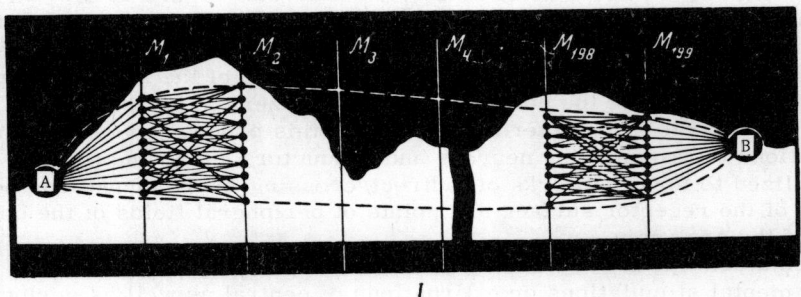

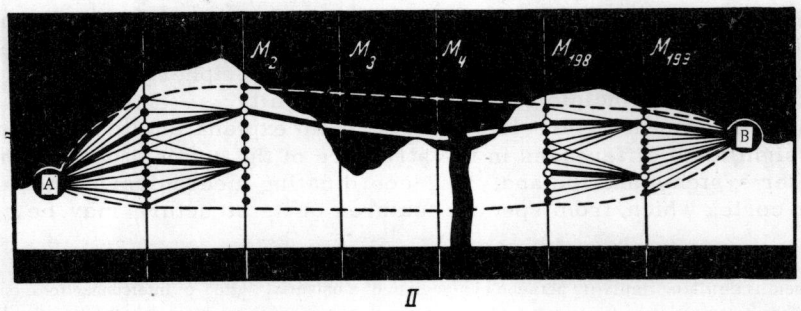

FIGURE 50. I. Diagram depicting the search for the optimal variant of a railway route between points A and B. With this diagram serving as the basis of route, the number of possible variants increases from district to district by geometric progression, reaching the astronomic number of 10^{200}.

II. Diagram depicting the solution of the same problem by means of an electronic computor and sequential analysis. The machine selects the optimal route from the innumerable possible connections between the districts. The possible connections are eliminated progressively until the separate sections of the route are connected in a single optimal line of the future main railway line.

The further differentiation of the structure of analyzer systems, as compared to the analyzing-coordinating mechanism, was conditioned by the following factors. In the progressive evolution of mammals, the functional interactions between analyzers become more and more varied; as a result, they become more intimately connected with each other and with their subcortical and, especially, cortical sections.

The development and differentiation of the entire system of opposite projected connections between sense organs and subcortical and cortical sections of the analyzer systems are associated with a corresponding development and differentiation of two-way connections between cortical zones of all analyzers represented in the cerebral hemispheres.

To the most highly differentiated cortical formations — related (according to I. N. Filimonov's classification) to the fully developed neocortex, to the systems of projectional (cortical-subcortical) and intercortical connections of the cortex (established through short-axon neurons) — is added a system of associating (intercortical or corticocortical) connections. The latter achieve a particularly high degree of development in higher mammals, the primates, and, among the primates, in man (Figures 52 and 55). With this, the general number of projecting and associating fibers going out from the cortex apparently exceeds the number of fibers entering the cortex. According to the data of D. A. Sholl* the visual cortex of the cat contains approximately 100,000 axons per mm; of these, 3/4 are efferent and only 1/4 afferent.

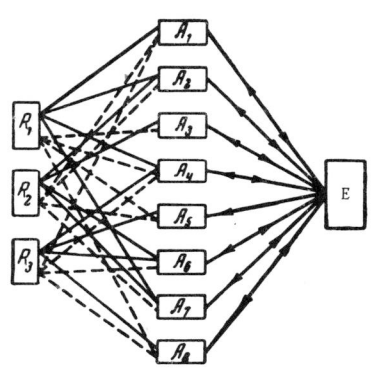

FIGURE 51. Diagram explaining the principle of action of a perceptron:

R — receptor units; A — associating units; E — effector units (from L. P. Kraizmer, 1962).

Through the system of associating connections the various cortical centers are able to act closely together and exchange stimulations. Thus the possibility of transmitting stimulations from the central field of the cortical zones to the peripheral ones through their associating connections was demonstrated by the method of neuronography in the skin and kinesthetic, as well as in the visual and auditory analyzers. The same method was also used to determine the presence of associating connections between different fields of the visual and auditory cortex. The formation of the system of associating connections has provided anatomical and physiological conditions assisting the most complex functional interconnections inside the cortical ending of a single analyzer, as well as between cortical endings of different analyzers.

One may accept the theory that the universal principle of mutual crossing over of pathways on the grid pattern, on which the entire CNS is based, also applies to the associating and projecting connections (Figure 53). An experimental physiological confirmation of this structural pattern of

---

* D. A. Sholl. Organization of the Cerebral Cortex. London. 1956.

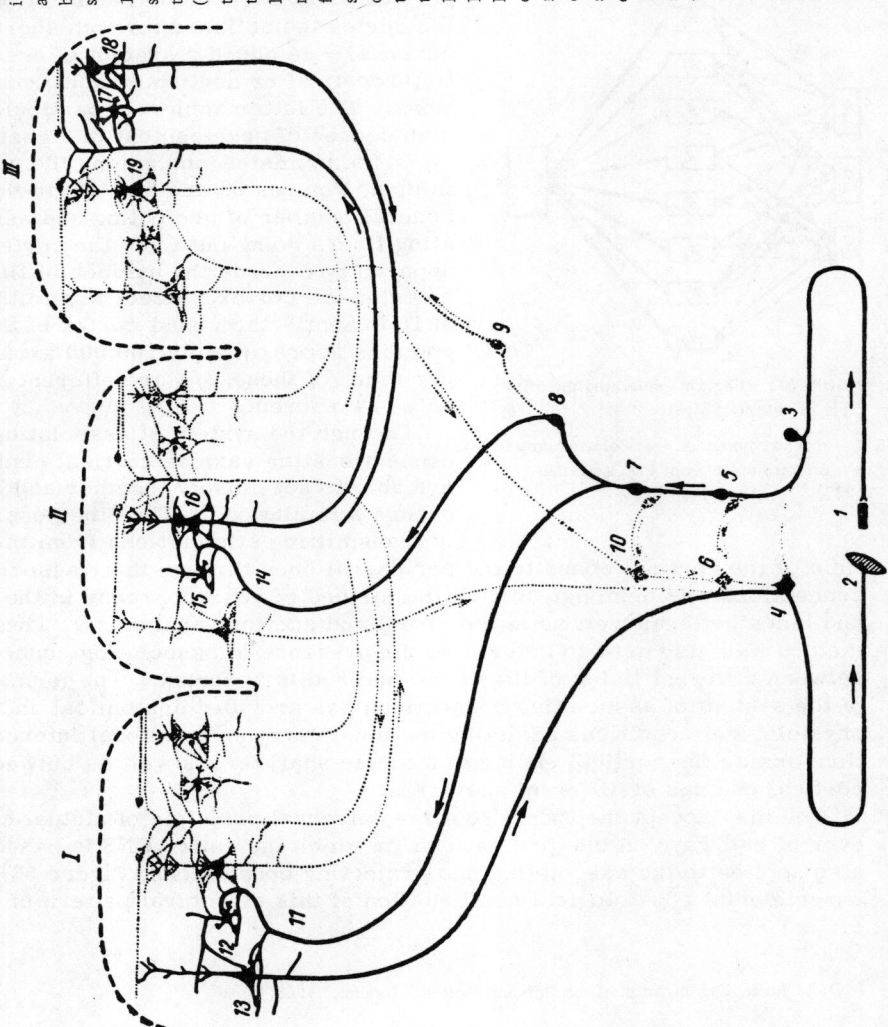

FIGURE 52. Diagram of topographic interrelations in the CNS of neuron complexes realizing intercortical projected (cortical-subcortical) and intercortical connections. Neurons included in any of the systems of connections are marked in black on the background of neurons of the other systems of connections, marked by a dotted line:

1 — receptor; 2 — effector; 3 — peripheral sensory neuron; 4 — effector (motor) neuron; 5,6 — transmitting neurons of the axial part of the CNS (spinal cord and brainstem); 7–10 — transmitting neurons of the supraaxial subcortical formations (nuclei of the optic thalamus and geniculate bodies, basal nuclei (ganglia) of the cerebral hemispheres); 11,14 — projected afferent fiber entering the cortex from a transmitting station in the subcortex; 13 — projected neuron of the cortex (pyramidal cell of layer V), initiating the cortical-motor pathway; 16 — associating neuron of the cortex (pyramidal cell of sublayer III_3); 18 — associating neuron of higher levels of the cortex (pyramidal cell of sublayers III_2 and III_1); 19 — associating afferent fiber entering the cortex; 12,15,17 — stellate neurons carrying out intercortical connections; I — central field of a nuclear zone of an analyzer; separated system of projected connections of the cortex (1–3–5–7–11–12–13–4–2). II — peripheral field of a nuclear zone of an analyzer; separated system of projected-associated connections of the cortex (1–3–5–7–8–14–15–16–19). III — field of a zone with overlapping of analyzers; separated system of inherent associating connections of the cortex (17–19). The diagram indicates consecutive extension of chains of neuron transmissions in transition from central to peripheral fields, and from those to zones with overlapping of analyzers (G.I. Poliakov, 1961).

associating connections in the human cerebral cortex is provided by recent electrophysiological studies by M. N. Livanov*; these studies are concerned with the problem of correlating analysis of the biopotentials of the brain in simultaneous multichannel leads from many points of the cortex. Figure 54 indicates the functional connections of the correlating cortical sections, constructed according to the principle of mutual crossing over, e.g., according to the grid pattern.

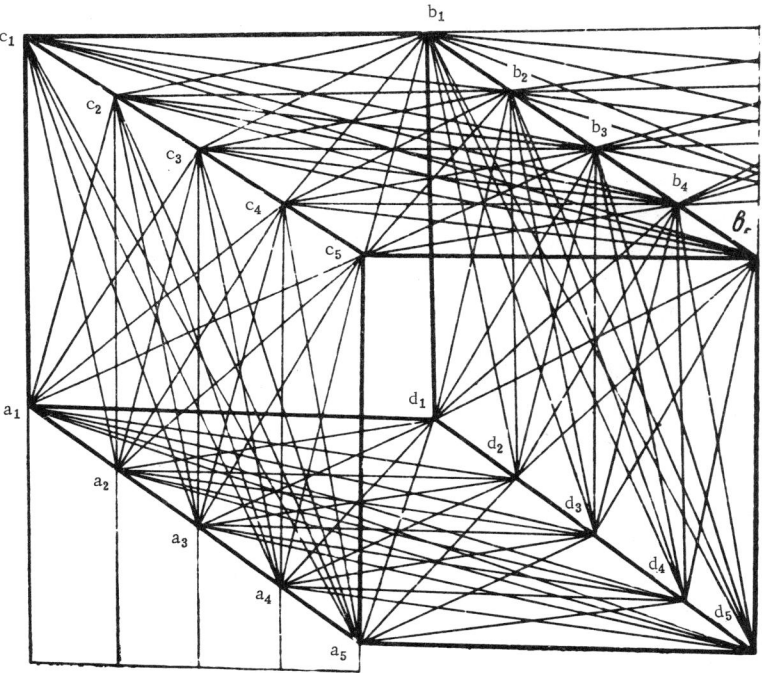

FIGURE 53. Universal diagram of the grid of interconnections, through which are realized both the functional unification (through projected connections) of transmitting points in the subcortex ($a_1 - a_5$) with corresponding points of the cortex ($b_1 - b_5$) and the functional unification (through associating connections) of different groups of neurons in the cortex (crossing-over grid of connections between $b_1 - b_5$ and $c_1 - c_5$). Note possibility of indirect connections of cortical points $c_1 - c_5$ with subcortical points $a_1 - a_5$, not only through transmissions $b_1 - b_5$ but also through additional transmissions in the subcortex $d_1 - d_5$ (so-called associating nuclei of the optic thalamus). The structure of transmissions in the brain depicted in the diagram constitutes a single entity.

* M.N. Livanov. Primenenie elektronno-vychislitel'noi tekhniki k analizu bioelektricheskikh protsessov golovnogo mozga (Use of Electronic Computer Techniques in Analysis of Bioelectric Processes of the Brain). — In: Biologicheskie aspekty kibernetiki. Moskva, Izdatel'stvo AN SSSR. 1962.

The separation of the cortex into architectonic layers and sublayers is based on the spatial demarcation inside the gray matter of complexes of neurons and zones with synaptic links adapted for completion of cortical-subcortical, intercortical and intracortical connections (see Figure 52). The differentiation — in the course of evolution of topographic correlations between neuron complexes related to different systems of connections of the cortex inside itself and with the subcortex — conditions the progressive differentiation of the cortex into various cytoarchitectonic areas, subareas, fields and subfields (see Figures 46 and 47).

Comparative analysis of data concerning differentiation of the CNS during ontophylogenesis allows one to conclude that a certain conformity exists in the development of all systems of connections uniting the different areas in the cortex with each other and with subcortical formations.

Generally this structural pattern may be defined as a successive extension of chains of neuron transmissions in systems of projecting and associating connections of the cortex, functioning in the process of transfer from the central fields to peripheral foci, and from these to the overlapping zones of analyzers (Figure 55, see also Figure 52). At the same time there is a separation of additional neuron transmissions in the cortical and subcortical sections of the analyzers.

Such additional groups of transmitting neurons in the cerebral cortex prove to be linked to peripheral fields and then to overlapping zones (Figure 55C, II and III), which could be considered as zones of merging and close functional interaction of elements of different analyzer functions. The anatomical expression of this process in the subcortical sections is the formation of so-called associating nuclei of the optic thalamus, in which are collected impulses from different analyzers (Figure 55B, 3 and 4). In certain sections of the optic thalamus there are groups of neurons which play the role of an association collector of the sum of sensory perceptions in the body (somatic receptors). The most important associational complex of the optic thalamus is the pulvinar, which functions as a body for the convergence of optic and auditory receptors. All these formations of the optic thalamus are joined by numerous bilateral (centripetal and centrifugal) connections with the overlapping zones of the cortical endings of the analyzers (distal and proximal parietal areas, temporo-parietal-occipital subarea).

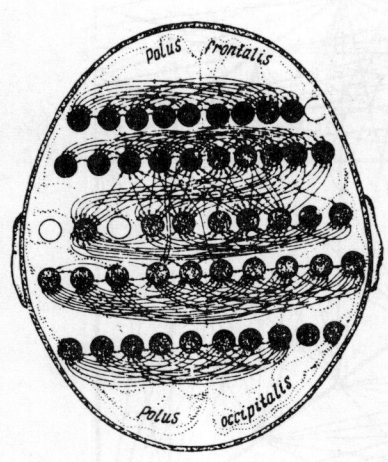

FIGURE 54. Temporary connections of points in the human brain during mental activity (solution of a logical problem). (After M.N. Livanov, 1962.)

One may thus conclude that the neuron structure undergoes the most extensive transformation at the centers of junctions and interpenetrations of qualitatively heterogeneous impulse currents. The overlapping zones in the cortical and associated subcortical areas of the analyzer systems, separated as a result of this process, are the most important integral part of the cerebral mechanisms which carry out various reactions to the most complex combinations of stimuli, and their interrelations.

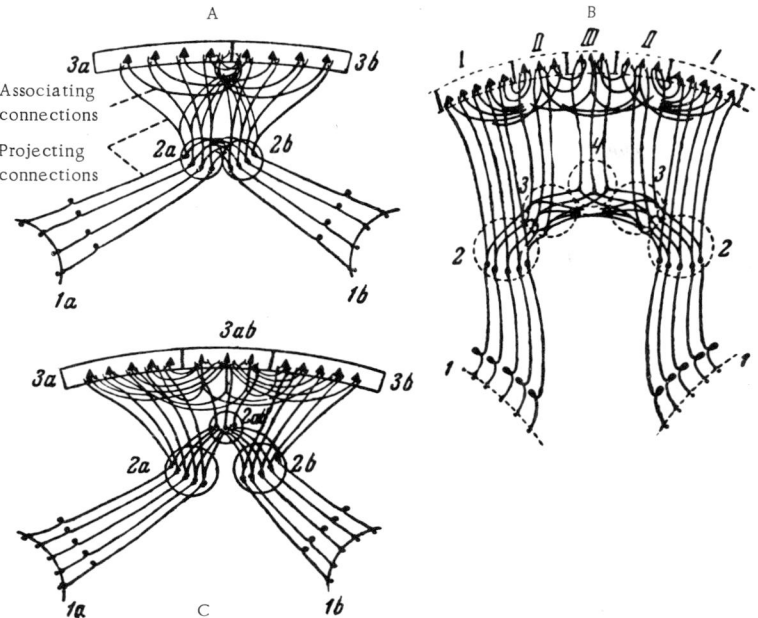

FIGURE 55. Diagrams depicting successive differentiation resulting from differentiation of functional interactions between analyzers, neuron transmissions and connections in the analyzer systems, in conformity with progressive structural differentiation in their cortical and subcortical transmitting stations:

A. 1a, 1b — peripheral receptor surfaces of analyzer systems; 2a, 2b — main transmitting ganglia in the lower subcortex (so-called relay nuclei of the optic thalamus), projecting into the nuclear zones of the analyzer systems in the cortex (3a, 3b). The diagram shows the beginning of formations of additional projecting and associating connections at junctional points and the interaction of cortical and subcortical components of both analyzers.
B. Same markings. Diagram shows the separation of additional impulse-transmitting stations in subcortical sections (so-called associating nuclei of the optic thalamus, 2ab) and in the cortex (overlapping zone of cortical endings of both analyzers, 3ab). Note that the main transmitting (relay) nuclei in subcortical parts (2a and 2b) project into nuclear zones, while the additional transmitting nuclei (2ab) are projected into the overlapping zone (3ab).
C. Diagram showing the further extension of chains of neuron transmissions in the cortical and subcortical sections of both analyzers, with corresponding differentiation of projecting and associating connections. 1 — peripheral receptor surfaces; 2, 3, 4 — ganglia of successive transmissions in subcortical sections (nuclei of optic thalamus and geniculate bodies). I — central fields; II — peripheral fields; III — overlapping zone. It is seen that the basic subcortical transmitting (relay) nuclei (2) are projected to the central fields, while the additional transmitting subcortical nuclei (3, 4) are projected to the peripheral fields and overlapping zone. (A – C, G. I. Poliakov, 1959 – 1961.)

The above-described structure of interconnections in the highest cerebral endings of the analyzer systems represents the physical basis of the diverse grades of transfer from actual sensory perceptions and impressions to abstract-logical forms of concepts of reality and behavior patterns.

CONCLUSION

The development of the structure of the brain during the course of animal evolution, enabling it to function as an organ of reflex activity, is expressed most strikingly by the increase in the number of successive levels of transmission of nerve impulses superimposed on each other. The range of adaptive possibilities of the organism in the initially poorly differentiated central nervous system expands; in addition there is a separation of a more and more complex morphological-physiological mechanism which participates in the formation of increasing numbers of branched chains of external and internal reactions, with the task of fulfilling the vitally important requirements of the organism. According to our concept, such mechanisms are part of the coordinating and analyzing-coordinating mechanisms and the analyzer systems.

The progressive development of reflex activity — caused by effects of dynamic conditions of life specific for the self-organizing biological system of the animal type — begins with the ability of the organism to effect coordinating responses to stimuli, i. e.; responses regulated in space and time and being of an adaptable character. We think that the coordinating mechanism, which becomes separated earliest in the phylogenesis of both invertebrates and vertebrates, is the morphophysiological basis of all vitally important autoregulations taking place inside the organism and appearing in its reactions to external stimuli in the process of constant adjustment to environmental changes.

According to our concept, the analyzers were formed in animal evolution as cerebral mechanisms with many additional "entries" to the coordinating mechanism and "exits" to the periphery of the body. The basic biological task of these central nervous formations is the realization of afferent syntheses inside the actual receptor sphere of the organism. This causes the formation of the necessary anatomical-physiological prerequisites for the realization of qualitatively higher forms of reprocessing of the total number of impulses entering the central nervous system, qualitatively superior to those of which the coordinating system is capable. This process is responsible for producing programs of response reactions ensuring an active adaptation to combinations of rapidly and diversely changing impulse stimuli.

The lowest developmental stage of analyzers, represented anatomically by the analyzing-coordinating mechanism, may be characterized as a structure through which a functional unification of different autoregulating adaptations of the entire organism is carried out. We define such a type of central nervous integration encompassing entire complexes of autoregulations, related mainly to the more elementary vital functions of the organism, as the function of autocontrol.

The highest developmental stage of analyzers is represented by the most complexly organized chains of neuron transmissions, i. e., the true analyzer systems. The highest (supraaxial) section of the analyzer systems, represented in vertebrates by the higher parts of the brain, are related to the most complexly integrated manifestations of reflex activity — those inborn and those acquired during life — from which the behavior of the organism as a whole is derived. We combine in the concept of autodirection the chains of instinctive inborn reactions associated with the phylogenetically more ancient cortical and subcortical formations, conditioned by the aggregation of biological requirements of the organism. We believe that phylogenetically newer cortical and subcortical formations associated with processes of accumulation of individual experience and reproductions of the most complex "cerebral models" of the environment, as well as production of corresponding behavior patterns, form the morphological-physiological basis of the function of direction in its true sense.

Stations of impulse transmissions, distributed along the axial part of the central nervous system and related to the analyzer systems, are constantly affected by opposite (centripetal and centrifugal) impulse currents, and have numerous collateral connections with groups of neurons of the coordinating and analyzing-coordinating mechanisms. We assume that on the basis of such a structure those functions of regulation and control are realized which, in keeping with our general theory, are of important auxiliary significance in the function of autoregulation and regulation.

We consider that evolutionally, the origin and development of analyzers represent a greater differentiation and a qualitative transformation of the main features of neuron structure, which are already present in the coordinating mechanism in a more elementary form. Analyzers, as well as the coordinating mechanism, are formed from the same basic types of neurons: efferent and special transmitting (intercalated or intermediate). The differentiation of the general structural pattern of neuron transmissions in analyzers, as compared to the coordinating mechanism, may be considered as a multiplication of parallel and successively linked elementary units of the coordinating mechanism; each such elementary fragment of the neuron network is formed by a certain combination of interconnections between afferent fibers and efferent and special transmitting neurons.

The special transmitting neurons are represented in the analyzers, together with reticular elements typical of the coordinating mechanism, mainly by elements with a finer and more complex differentiation — short-axon neurons. The latter reach a particularly distinct development in the highest brain endings of the analyzer systems. With the active participation of this type of neuron, the coordination of interactions between the separate groups of efferent neurons in the chains of transmissions is carried out; the latter are concerned with the transfer and reprocessing of impulses specific for each analyzer system. The short-axon neurons, together with the returning collaterals of axons of efferent neurons, play quite a significant role in the completion of impulse circuits in certain constellations of neurons, localized at the same or at different levels of the CNS. Because of a corresponding organization of interconnections between afferent fibers and efferent and special transmitting neurons, optimal conditions are ensured for fine discrimination and adequate interpretation of separate impulse stimuli and their complexes in space-time relationships. This type of structure is particularly valuable for retention of excitation traces of stimuli which had acted on the organism before, and for their connection with current reactions. The cerebral cortex contains particularly numerous short-axon neurons (stellate cells) which are variously differentiated as to the form and specific structure of their dendritic and axonal branchings; this supports our hypothesis of their important role in cortical processes of analysis and synthesis of external and internal impulses.

With the formation of a fully developed neocortex as it appears in mammals, the highest cerebral endings of the analyzer systems and the organization of different forms of interneuron connections attain the highest degree of differentiation, as compared to less developed levels of the CNS. In these cortical formations we have noted terminal contacts of axon ramifications with bodies and initial sections of dendrites of nerve cells adapted mainly for direct effects of certain neurons on others; in addition there are numerous contacts of the tangential type, established between ramifications of axons and lateral outgrowths ("spines"), acting on dendrites of efferent neurons (pyramidal and spindle-shaped cells). We assume that by means of the tangential contacts indirect effects on the functional condition of the given efferent neuron are realized through numerous other neurons. The particularly significant development of this type of contact in the cerebral cortex may, from our point of view, serve as a morphological confirmation of the extensive functional range of cortical neurons.

The stellate cells (as well as the reticular neurons), unlike the efferent long-axon neurons, are, with all the distinct features of their fine structure and connections, specialized mainly for the establishment of terminal contacts with other neurons. The morphological facts correspond to our present concepts of the role of the special transmitting neurons in the most delicate processes of differentiation and integration of stimuli entering the cerebral cortex and circulating in its gray matter.

Our hypothesis on the origin of the natural network of neurons allows us to formulate a single synthetic concept concerning the nature of progressive differentiation of neuron structure in animal evolution. Our concept is based on the structural pattern of connections between different levels of impulse transmissions along the pathways traversed by the analyzers, including the crossing over, according to the grid pattern, from their peripheral origins to the highest cortical endings. In principle, this type of structure provides a connection, through a series of intermediate transmissions in the distal and proximal subcortical areas, between any point of the sensory receptor surface of the analyzer at the periphery of the body with any point of the cortical zone of an analyzer.

Following this concept, the differentiation of the analyzer-system structure during evolutionary progress may be shown to undergo a gradual separation from the initially uniform "diffuse" grid of interconnections of neuron-transmission chains, becoming more and more highly specialized for the transfer of impulse currents of varying types. At the same time, there is a separation in the rod part of the trunk system of the analyzer, adjusted to the shortest and most direct projections from the periphery to the central field of the nuclear zone of the analyzer in the cerebral cortex, with a relatively small number of intermediate transmissions. Through such projections, organized according to the somatotopic principle, the most concentrated currents of "specific" impulses corresponding to a certain modality are transferred; this ensures a high capacity for "authorized" activities of the analyzer system, providing it with fine discriminating ability concerning various aspects of impulse stimuli.

In the process of differentiation of the analytical synthetic activity in the analyzer systems both relatively short and direct pathways of impulse transmissions and also longer chains of neurons with a large number of intermediate transmissions become distinct, connecting elements of the receptor surface with peripheral fields of nuclear zones of cortical analyzers. This part of the structure of the analyzer system provides the ability to carry out the more complexly related interaction between groups of receptors and corresponding complexes of cortical neurons; impulses originating at the same point of the receptor surface can thus reach different points of the cortex; impulses from different parts of the receptor surface may also converge at different points of the cortex. Such a pattern of interconnections provides the physiological prerequisites for various types of integration of fine-discrimination impulse stimuli.

The anatomical substrate of increasing differentiation of functional relations between analyzer systems in mammals is the formation of overlapping zones of analyzer endings in the cortex, as well as further structural differentiation of nuclear zones of analyzers in the central and peripheral fields.

Unlike the nuclear zones, which can be characterized as areas of concentration of elements of definite modality, specific for the given analyzer, the overlapping zones represent closely distributed collections of elements of different analyzers. These "internuclear" zones — represented by fields in the distal and proximal parietal areas, the temporo-parietal-occipital subarea and the frontal area — achieve their highest degree of development in primates, and among the primates, in man. These cortical formations are related to the most generalized forms of analytic-synthetic activity which are formed on the basis of complex interactions of elements of different analytical functions. These complex processes and the functional organization of the brain are expressed in primates by the marked development of associating connections in the cortex; they provide contact of cortical zones of different analyzers with each other, with other analyzers, and with internuclear overlapping zones.

The progressive differentiation of nuclear zones in the central and peripheral fields, and the concomitant separations of overlapping zones in the cerebral cortex, are also associated with a corresponding reorganization of neuron transmissions in the proximal subcortex, in the form of additional formations to the relay nuclei, the so-called associating nuclei of the optic thalamus.

There is a definite correlation between the degree of development of all systems of connections, and their integrating action on different parts of the cerebral cortex, involving themselves and the subcortical formations. This structural pattern may be described as a successive extension of neuron-transmission chains in the cortical systems of projection and association connections during the transfer from central fields of nuclear zones to peripheral ones, and from these to overlapping zones of analyzers. At the same time, additional neuron transmissions are delineated in cortical and subcortical sections of the analyzers.

In summary one may state that present data concerning the architecture, neuron structure and connections of the CNS allow some general deductions to be made, although their functional significance is still not entirely clear. A comparative analysis of the origin, development and differentiation of these mechanisms in animal evolution brings us closer to the solution of the cardinal question posed by Pavlov: what is the fine structure of the analyzers, and how do their various components interact?

EXPLANATORY LIST OF ABBREVIATED NAMES OF USSR INSTITUTIONS APPEARING IN REFERENCES IN THIS TEXT

Abbreviation	Full name (transliterated)	Translation
AMN SSSR	Akademiya meditsinskikh nauk SSSR	Academy of Medical Sciences of the USSR
AN SSSR	Akademiya nauk SSSR	Academy of Sciences of the USSR
APN SSSR	Akademiya pedagogicheskikh nauk SSSR	Academy of Pedagogical Sciences of the USSR
LGU	Leningradskii gosudarstvennyi universitet	Leningrad State University
MGU	Moskovskii gosudarstvennyi universitet	Moscow State University